Pain

What Psychiatrists
Need to Know

Review of Psychiatry Series
John M. Oldman, M.D., and
Michelle B. Riba, M.D.
Series Editors

Pain

What Psychiatrists Need to Know

EDITED BY

Mary Jane Massie, M.D.

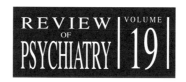

REVIEW OF PSYCHIATRY — VOLUME 19

No. 2

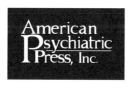

American Psychiatric Press, Inc.

Washington, DC
London, England

Copyright © 2000 American Psychiatric Press, Inc.

04   03   02   01   5   4   3   2

ALL RIGHTS RESERVED

Manufactured in the United States of America on acid-free paper
First Edition

American Psychiatric Press, Inc.
1400 K Street, NW
Washington, DC 20005
www.appi.org

The correct citation for this book is

> Massie MJ (ed.): *Pain: What Psychiatrists Need to Know* (Review of Psychiatry Series, Vol. 19, No. 2; Oldham JM and Riba MB, series eds.). Washington, DC, American Psychiatric Press, 2000

Library of Congress Cataloging-in-Publication Data
Pain : what psychiatrists need to know / edited by Mary Jane Massie.
      p. ; cm. — (Review of psychiatry ; v. 19, no. 2)
    Includes bibliographical references and index.
    ISBN 0-88048-173-0 (alk. paper)
    1. Pain. 2. Psychiatry. I. Massie, Mary Jane. II. Review of psychiatry
series ; v. 19, 2
    [DNLM: 1. Chronic Disease. 2. Pain. 3. Psychotherapy—methods.
WL 704 P14793 2000]
RB127.P365 2000
616´.0472—dc21

                                                                00-023877

British Library Cataloguing in Publication Data
A CIP record is available from the British Library.

Review of Psychiatry Series ISSN 1041-5882

Contents

Contributors

Augusto Caraceni, M.D.
Chief, Neurology Unit, Rehabilitation and Palliative Care Unit, Department of Anesthesia and Critical Care, National Cancer Institute, Milan, Italy

Lisa Chertkov, M.D.
Clinical Fellow, Department of Psychiatry and Behavioral Sciences, Memorial Sloan-Kettering Cancer Center, New York, New York

Andrea Cheville, M.D.
Assistant Professor of Rehabilitation Medicine, Director, cancer Rehabilitation, Department of Rehabilitation Medicine, University of Pennsylvania Health Care System, Philadelphia, Pennsylvania

Stewart B. Fleishman, M.D.
Director, Cancer Supportive Services, Cancer Center, Beth Israel Medical Center, New York, New York, Associate Clinical Professor of Psychiatry, Albert Einstein College of Medicine, Bronx, New York

Barbara Kamholz, M.D.
Clinical Assistant Professor, Department of Psychiatry, University of Michigan Medical Center, Chief, Psychiatry Consultation Services, V. A. Ann Arbor Hill System, Ann Arbor, Michigan

Mary Jane Massie, M.D.
Attending Psychiatrist and Director, Barbara White Fishman Center for Psychological Counseling, Memorial Sloan-Kettering Cancer Center, Professor of Clinical Psychiatry, Joan and Sanford I. Weill Medical College of Cornell University, New York, New York

Philip R. Muskin, M.D.
Chief, Consultation Liaison Psychiatry Service, Department of Psychiatry, Columbia Presbyterian Hospital of the New York Presbyterian Medical Center, Associate Professor of Clinical Psychiatry, Columbia University, College of Physicians and Surgeons, New York, New York

John M. Oldham, M.D.
Director, New York State Psychiatric Institute; Dollard Professor and Acting Chairman, Department of Psychiatry, Columbia University College of Physicians and Surgeons, New York, New York

Russell K. Portenoy, M.D.
Chairman, Department of Pain Medicine and Palliative Care, Beth Israel Medical Center, New York, New York, Professor of Neurology, Albert Einstein College of Medicine, Bronx, New York

Michelle B. Riba, M.D.
Clinical Associate Professor of Psychiatry and Associate Chair for Education and Academic Affairs, Department of Psychiatry, University of Michigan Health System, Ann Arbor, Michigan

Randy S. Roth, Ph.D.
Clinical Assistant Professor, Departments of Physical Medicine and Rehabilitation, Anesthesiology, and Psychology, Adjunct Lecturer, Department of Psychology, University of Michigan Health System, Ann Arbor, Michigan

Introduction to the Review of Psychiatry Series

John M. Oldham, M.D.,
Michelle B. Riba, M.D., Series Editors

2000 REVIEW OF PSYCHIATRY SERIES TITLES

- *Learning Disabilities: Implications for Psychiatric Treatment*
  EDITED BY LAURENCE L. GREENHILL, M.D.
- *Psychotherapy for Personality Disorders*
  EDITED BY JOHN G. GUNDERSON, M.D., AND GLEN O. GABBARD, M.D.
- *Ethnicity and Psychopharmacology*
  EDITED BY PEDRO RUIZ, M.D.
- *Complementary and Alternative Medicine and Psychiatry*
  EDITED BY PHILIP R. MUSKIN, M.D.
- *Pain: What Psychiatrists Need to Know*
  EDITED BY MARY JANE MASSIE, M.D.

The advances in knowledge in the field of psychiatry and the neurosciences in the last century can easily be described as breathtaking. As we embark on a new century and a new millennium, we felt that it would be appropriate for the 2000 Review of Psychiatry Series monographs to take stock of the state of that knowledge at the interface between normality and pathology. Although there may be nothing new under the sun, we are learning more about not-so-new things, such as how we grow and develop; who we are; how to differentiate between just being different from one another and being ill; how to recognize, treat, and perhaps prevent illness; how to identify our unique vulnerabilities; and how to deal with the inevitable stress and pain that await each of us.

In the early years of life, for example, how can we tell whether a particular child is just rowdier, less intelligent, or more adventuresome than another child—or is, instead, a child with a learning or behavior disorder? Clearly, the distinction is crucial, because newer and better treatments that now exist for early-onset disorders can smooth the path and enhance the chances for a solid future for children with such disorders. Yet, inappropriately labeling and treating a rambunctious but normal child can create problems rather than solve them. Greenhill and colleagues guide us through these waters, illustrating that a highly sophisticated methodology has been developed to make this distinction with accuracy, and that effective treatments and interventions are now at hand.

Once we have successfully navigated our way into early adulthood, we are supposed to have a pretty good idea (so the advice books say) of who we are. Of course, this stage of development does not come easy, nor at the same time, for all. Again, a challenge presents itself—that is, to differentiate between widely disparate varieties of temperament and character and when extremes of personality traits and styles should be recognized as disorders. And even when traits are so extreme that little dispute exists that a disorder is present, does that disorder represent who the person is, or is it something the individual either inherited or developed and might be able to overcome? In the fifth century B.C., Hippocrates described different personality types that he proposed were correlated with specific "body humors"; this ancient principle remains quite relevant, though the body humors of today are neurotransmitters. How low CNS serotonin levels need to be, for example, to produce disordered impulsivity is still being determined, yet new symptom-targeted treatment of such conditions with SSRIs is now well accepted. What has been at risk as the neurobiology of personality disorders has become increasingly understood is the continued recognition of the importance of psychosocial treatments for these disorders. Gunderson and Gabbard and their colleagues review the surprisingly robust evidence for the effectiveness of these approaches, including new uses and types of cognitive-behavioral and psychoeducational methods.

It is not just differences in personality that distinguish us from one another. Particularly in our new world of global communication and population migration, ethnic and cultural differences are more often part of life in our own neighborhoods than just exotic and unfamiliar aspects of faraway lands. Despite great strides overcoming fears and prejudices, much work remains to be done. At the same time, we must learn more about ways that we are different (not better or worse) genetically and biologically, because uninformed ignorance of these differences leads to unacceptable risks. Ruiz and colleagues carefully present what we now know and do not know about ethnicity and its effects on pharmacokinetics and pharmacodynamics.

An explosion of interest in and information about wellness—not just illness—surrounds us. How to achieve and sustain a healthy lifestyle, how to enhance successful aging, and how to benefit from "natural" remedies saturate the media. Ironically, although this seems to be a new phenomenon, the principles of complementary or alternative medicine are ancient. Some of our oldest and most widely used medications are derived from plants and herbs, and Eastern medicine has for centuries relied on concepts of harmony, relaxation, and meditation. Again, as the world shrinks, we are obligated to be open to ideas that may be new to us but not to others and to carefully evaluate their utility. Muskin and colleagues present a careful analysis of the most familiar and important components of complementary and alternative medicine, presenting a substantial database of information, along with tutorials on non-Western (hence nontraditional to us) concepts and beliefs.

Like it or not, life presents us with stress and pain. Pain management has not typically figured into mainstream psychiatric training or practice (with the exception of consultation-liaison psychiatry), yet it figures prominently in the lives of us all. Massie and colleagues provide us with a primer on what psychiatrists should know about the subject, and there is a great deal indeed that we should know.

Many other interfaces exist between psychiatry as a field of medicine, defining and treating psychiatric illnesses, and the rest of medicine—and between psychiatry and the many paths of the life cycle. These considerations are, we believe, among our top priorities as we begin the new millennium, and these volumes provide an in-depth review of some of the most important ones.

Foreword

Mary Jane Massie, M.D.

Chronic pain is a critical issue in health care today. Beyond the untold personal suffering, the cost in lost workdays and health care dollars is enormous. At any given moment, half of all Americans will have experienced some pain within the previous 2 weeks. Disabling, chronic, nonmalignant pain affects about 34 million people (Leitman and Binnisk Unni 1994). In almost 16% of the households in America, at least one person has severe chronic pain, and research indicates that the number of people with chronic pain in the United States is increasing. For example, the Michigan Pain Study (1997) found that 20% of a random sample of 1,500 adults have some form of chronic or recurrent pain.

The total annual cost of pain in the United States (including medical expenses, lost income, and lost productivity) is estimated to exceed $100 billion (Bonica 1980). Annual absenteeism from work resulting from pain exceeds 50 million days per year and approximately 170 million people-days of pain-related, short-term work disability (Schwartz 1999). Thus, pain poses a critical challenge to our society and to the clinician as we struggle to better understand chronic pain and to more effectively treat the suffering endured by so many.

Back pain, chronic abdominal and pelvic pain, migraine headaches, and fibromyalgia each affect many people, taking a toll on personal and professional lives, and costing countless dollars for traditional and alternative therapies. Among the different types of nonmalignant pain, acute low back pain is predominant, affecting 70%–80% of adults at some time in their lives (Daltroy et al. 1997). Short-term bed rest is often self-prescribed for this acute, usually self-limited condition. In recent years, however, evidence indicating the lack of effectiveness of bed rest for low back pain and sciatica has accumulated. Most acute low back pain improves with watchful waiting (Deyo et al. 1986; Malmivaara et al. 1995; Vroomen 1999).

Chronic low back pain occurs in 3% of the population and is one of the most frequent reasons that patients seek the aid of primary care physicians. It is the second most common reason for missed workdays (Nachemson 1992). In fact, back symptoms are the most common cause of disability in the United States for persons younger than 45 years (Rosomoff and Rosomoff 1999). Despite extensive research, no consensus has evolved about prevention, diagnosis, and treatment of chronic low back pain. The consequences, however, of chronic back pain are often described by patients as demoralization and depressive symptoms. In fact, the reported prevalence of depression in individuals with chronic low back pain is three to four times that observed in the general population, although the interpretation of this increased prevalence is controversial (Sullivan et al. 1992).

Chronic abdominal and pelvic pain similarly affects a substantial percentage of the population, especially women. A recent study showed that 11% of primary care visits were for abdominal pain symptoms (Kroenke 1991). Walker and colleagues (1991) showed that among 650 women attending two ambulatory care clinics, 38% reported persistent lower abdominal pain of greater than 6 months' duration at some time in their lives. Controversy also exists about the etiology of psychological symptoms in individuals with chronic abdominal and pelvic pain and other frequently observed pain problems in ambulatory care clinics.

Migraine headache, another common chronic pain disorder, affects approximately 17% of the women and 6% of the men in the United States each year (Stewart et al. 1994). The total number of sick days attributed to migraines was estimated at 1.4 million days, at a total annual cost of $185.4 million. Despite the high prevalence of comorbid psychiatric disorders (depression, sleep disturbance, obsessive-compulsive disorder, bipolar disorder, anxiety disorders, and chemical dependence) in patients with migraines, and the high cost of suffering and impaired function, more than 90% of those with a headache disorder have never been to a specialist (Saper 1999).

Fibromyalgia, another controversial chronic pain disorder, has been the subject of extensive popular and medical debate about its etiology, parameters, psychological connections, and treatment. Most patients who have fibromyalgia complain of multiple symptoms, such as achiness, burning pain, severe fatigue, sleep disorder, irritable bowel syndrome, headaches, temporomandibular joint pain, multiple chemical sensitivity syndrome, chest pain, morning stiffness, and painful menstrual periods. Exploration of the etiology and treatment of fibromyalgia, as in many of the other chronic pain disorders, has raised many questions about psychiatric comorbidity and the role of psychotropic medications in the treatment of chronic pain. In their search for relief, patients turn to traditional biomedical care and to alternatives ranging from chiropractors to herbal remedies.

The increasing prevalence of chronic pain in the United States has led to reformulations of the definition of pain in an effort to more fully encompass its biopsychosocial features and to provide for a more accurate description of symptoms and targeted interventions. Pain is increasingly understood as an integrated cognitive, psychological, and sensory experience, not simply as neurological phenomena. This more comprehensive model has led to the exploration of new and combined treatment modalities. The treatments for chronic pain are categorized as pharmacological, anesthesiological, surgical, neurostimulatory, physiatric, psychological, and complementary (see Caraceni, Cheville, and Portenoy, Chapter 2, in this volume). Psychological strategies for the treatment of pain are increasingly being used and proven effective, and many pain patients find them an appealing alternative to drug therapy. These treatment modalities encompass educational programs, cognitive-behavioral therapy, and psychotherapy, including group therapy, biofeedback, hypnosis, exercise, relaxation, and distraction techniques.

But which patients should receive psychological treatments? All? Those who "fail" one, two, or three biomedical approaches? Those who "look" psychiatrically impaired? Over the last three decades, as the number of studies of the prevalence of psychiatric disorders in individuals with many medical illnesses has increased, research groups have attempted to provide better data on pain and comorbid psychiatric disorders and symptoms. Others have recently reviewed the topic of comorbid pain and psychiatric disorders (Fishbain 1999; Koenig and Clarke 1996).

required for the inciting problem to resolve. Alternatively, chronic pain is associated with a lesion that is not expected to heal. The patient typically has few pain behaviors and no sympathetic hyperactivity. Sleep disturbance is very common, and some patients develop other vegetative signs, such as lassitude or anorexia. Patients often describe some combination of depressed mood, anxiety, and irritability (Romano and Turner 1985).

Temporal profiles vary markedly among patients with chronic pain. Most patients have waxing and waning pain punctuated by pain-free intervals. Even those with continuous pain report large fluctuations in the severity of pain. Some have severe exacerbations of pain that are perceived as distinct from the baseline pain. In a survey of patients with cancer, for example, almost two-thirds reported transient episodes of severe "breakthrough" pain; these episodes varied greatly in duration, frequency, and quality (Portenoy and Hagen 1990; Portenoy et al. 1999).

The temporal profile of the pain may be important in the development of a therapeutic approach to the patient. For example, prominent breakthrough pain suggests several specific strategies, such as the use of a short-acting analgesic administered in a preemptive fashion.

Pain Intensity

Measurement of pain severity is an essential part of the pain assessment. Valid measurement can be performed with simple unidimensional scales or multidimensional questionnaires. The choice of a particular method in clinical practice is probably less important than its systematic application repeatedly over time (Au et al. 1994). The clinician should select a method and incorporate its use into the clinical routine, obtaining the measurement in the same manner each time.

Regardless of the scale, both the time frame of assessment and the clinical context must be defined (Chapman et al. 1985). With chronic pain, it may be useful to inquire about pain during the "past month" and obtain separate measurements for pain "on average," pain "at its least," and pain "at its worst." A measurement rating of pain intensity "right now" sometimes offers another useful perspective. Patients with acute pain usually are asked to rate their pain "right now" and also may be asked to indicate the average intensity during a fixed time, such as the past day.

A categorical verbal rating scale ("none," "mild," "moderate," "severe") is the simplest measure. Most patients also find an 11-point numerical scale ("On a scale of 0 to 10, where 0 is no pain and 10 is the worst pain imaginable, how severe is your pain right now?") understandable. Either of these scales can be applied at the bedside as a verbal query (response recorded by the nurse) or a written question. The patient can use the identical scale at home as part of a daily pain diary, in which the intensity of pain can be recorded at fixed times during the day (e.g., one to three times per day). Empirical data indicate that three daily assessments will provide very accurate information about the pain experience of patients with chronic nonmalignant pain (Jensen and McFarland 1993). If a notation about activity and drug use is recorded at the same time as a pain rating, the diary can be a very useful technique for clarifying the relations among pain, activity, and the effect of treatment.

Another valid approach for pain measurement is a visual analogue scale (VAS) (Banos et al. 1989). This scale typically uses a 10-cm line, anchored at one end by the descriptor "no pain" or "least possible pain" and anchored at the other end by "worst possible pain." The patient marks the line at the point that best describes the pain intensity, and the distance from the left end is used as the pain measurement.

The scores on the various pain intensity scales are highly correlated (De Conno et al. 1994; Price 1988). Several studies have reported that the VAS is more sensitive than other scales to variations in pain intensity over time, but this does not necessarily translate into a clinically relevant difference (Wirth and Van Buren 1971). Some patients find the VAS more difficult to understand than either verbal categorical or numerical scales.

Multidimensional pain scales have been developed to quantitate and characterize various aspects of the pain. Sensory and affective pain descriptors can be distinguished (Melzack 1975), and pain-related functional impairment can be separated from pain intensity (Daut et al. 1983). These instruments are longer and generally are used in clinical research.

Pain Location

Most patients have little difficulty describing the regions of the body affected by the pain. For those who do have difficulty, body maps may be useful (Margoles 1983). Pain syndromes may be focal (i.e., confined to an isolated site), multifocal, or generalized. This distinction is clinically relevant because treatment approaches may vary depending on pain distribution. For example, nerve blocks usually are considered only if the pain is focal.

As part of this assessment, the clinician should ask the patient whether the pain is superficial or deep. This distinction can be made more easily by likening the pain to a "muscle cramp," "sunburn," or "toothache."

Pain may be experienced superficial to the underlying etiology (sometimes also termed a *focal* pain) or may be referred to a region distant from this site. Lesions involving virtually any structure, whether somatic, visceral, or neural, can give rise to referred pain. Recognition of pain referral patterns is essential to formulate a hypothesis concerning the etiology or pathophysiology of the pain.

The pain referral patterns from lesions affecting visceral structures are widely recognized. Cardiac ischemia can cause pain in the left shoulder, arm, or jaw. Involvement of the diaphragm may refer pain to the cap of the ipsilateral shoulder, and disease in the region of the porta hepatis may refer pain to the ipsilateral scapula.

Referred pain from neurological lesions may pose a more significant diagnostic challenge. An injured nerve can cause focal pain superficial to the site of injury or refer pain anywhere in the dermatome innervated by the nerve. Toe pain can herald a sciatic mononeuropathy, a lumbosacral plexopathy, or an L5 or S1 radiculopathy. These lesions also can produce pain superficial to the site of injury, just as median nerve entrapment in the carpal tunnel often presents as aching in the wrist. Although back pain is suggestive of a root lesion, it is not specific, and painful radiculopathy can occur entirely without back pain.

In some cases, pain caused by a focal nerve injury may be referred outside the confines of a single dermatome or peripheral nerve distribution. For example, patients with median nerve entrapment at the wrist may feel a diffuse aching in the shoulder, upper arm, or full hand or palm (Torebjork et al. 1984).

Injury to brachial or lumbosacral plexuses can produce pain with varying distributions. Although the pain is often segmental (e.g., tumor involvement of the brachial plexus often causes symptoms of a C8-T1 radiculopathy), it may be more diffuse and span several dermatomes.

Polyneuropathy usually produces pain that begins in both feet and may gradually ascend proximally to involve the distal legs. As the disease progresses, these sensations may involve the hands bilaterally ("stocking-glove" distribution).

The topography of neuropathic pain associated with lesions of the central nervous system is particularly variable. Depending on the level of injury, pain related to a spinal cord lesion may be experienced as dysesthesias in the torso or in one or more extremities. In some patients, these lesions generate symmetrical pain in the feet and distal legs that can mimic painful polyneuropathy. Segmental pain alone, which mimics nerve root compression, may be caused by a lesion of the root entry zone inside the spinal cord. A lesion in the brain stem may cause "crossed" dysesthesias involving the ipsilateral face and contralateral body, and a more rostral lesion can cause either chronic pain in the entire contralateral hemibody or a highly focal pain in one site. Thus, remarkably, a chronic pain in the toe could even be the result of a lesion in the contralateral cerebral cortex.

Knowledge of the classic pain distribution patterns associated with neurological injury may provide guidance in localizing a lesion. Conversely, failure to recognize these patterns can lead to unnecessary delay in diagnosis.

Exacerbating and Alleviating Factors

Clarification of the factors that exacerbate or alleviate pain may help to define its etiology or pathophysiology and suggest treatment strategies. Pain with postures or movements may suggest structural disease at specific sites. For example, shoulder pain elicited with abduction beyond 90 degrees with the arm in an internally rotated position is indicative of rotator cuff tendonitis. Discogenic back pain usually is relieved by rest and increased by

Pain that is perceived to be sustained by abnormal somatosensory processing in the peripheral or central nervous system is termed *neuropathic* pain. In some cases, these pains appear to have a persistent peripheral "generator" (painful peripheral mono- or polyneuropathies). Painful peripheral mononeuropathy may involve nerve entrapment (e.g., carpal tunnel syndrome), neuroma formation after nerve injury (e.g., stump pain), nerve inflammation (e.g., herpes zoster), or other processes. Painful polyneuropathies may be related to any of a very large number of disease processes or toxic insults.

Other types of neuropathic pains have a generator in the central nervous system (also termed *deafferentation pains*) or are believed to be partially or wholly sustained by efferent activity in the sympathetic nervous system (labeled *sympathetically maintained* pains). Deafferentation pains may be caused by injury to either peripheral nerves (such as occurs in phantom pain) or the brain or spinal cord itself. Sympathetically maintained pains, which are most commonly identified among patients with the clinical syndromes of reflex sympathetic dystrophy and causalgia, may be initiated by injury to nerves or somatic structures.

Neuropathic pain may be described as unfamiliar, burning, or shocklike (Gracely and Kwilosz 1988). These descriptors are not specific, however. Similar burning pain also occurs with skin inflammation or a first-degree burn, in which case it is best categorized as a somatic nociceptive pain. Moreover, some patients with neuropathic pain, such as those with radiculopathy from discogenic disease, commonly describe pain in familiar terms, such as aching and throbbing.

Some patients have strong evidence of a predominating psychological contribution to the pain. Pain specialists often refer generically to these pains as *psychogenic*. These patients can also be more specifically categorized in terms of the somatoform disorders described in DSM-IV (American Psychiatric Association 1994).

These pathophysiological constructs have important therapeutic implications. Various nontraditional analgesics, such as anticonvulsants and oral local anesthestics, may be considered for neuropathic pain. Although inferred pathophysiology alone should not be used to select patients for an opioid trial, neuropathic pain appears to be relatively less responsive to opioids than nociceptive pain (Portenoy et al. 1990; Turk and Rudy 1990). Nociceptive pain is also generally believed to be more responsive than other types of pain to invasive therapies designed to isolate the painful part, such as cordotomy.

An integration of a medical-physical classification, such as the pathophysiological constructs, and a psychosocial and behavioral classification ultimately may be the most useful method of categorizing patients with chronic pain. This so-called polydiagnostic approach has been explored (Kerns et al. 1985; Turk and Rudy 1988) and is a promising area for further study.

Syndromic Classification

Syndrome identification can direct further assessment of the pain, suggest the likely etiology, or predict the efficacy of a therapeutic approach. The utility of disease-specific pain syndromes in the management of selected populations, such as those with cancer, is well established (Gonzales et al. 1991).

Some syndromic labels are used commonly but are vague and must be applied with caution. For example, the term *chronic non-malignant pain syndrome,* which appears at first glance to refer to any type of persistent pain, is actually applied conventionally to patients who have poorly controlled pain that is disproportionate to any evident pathology and is associated with a high level of disability and psychological disturbance. Thus, this label implies the existence of significant comorbid psychological and behavioral problems and, as such, could be unnecessarily stigmatizing. In a similar manner, potentially stigmatizing implications have been attached to a variety of site-specific terms, such as *atypical facial pain, failed low back syndrome, chronic tension headache,* and *chronic pelvic pain of unknown etiology.* When physicians apply these terms, they should provide additional explanation of the factors that may be contributing to the pain and specifically indicate the existence of comorbidities.

Evaluation of Associated Phenomena

The evaluation of the patient's medical status, physical impairments, psychological adjustment, comorbid psychiatric disorders, vocational viability, and social functioning is critical in a comprehensive pain assessment. The degree of physical impairment and associated physical and psychosocial disability is the strongest indicator of the need for a specialized approach to pain management, typically one that uses a multimodality strategy implemented by an interdisciplinary team.

Assessing Physical and Psychosocial Functioning

Functional deficits secondary to effects of physical impairments (such as weakness or sensory loss) must be distinguished from the effect of unrelieved pain or consequences of pain therapy. The interactions among pain, pain-related disability, and other psychological and psychiatric concerns, including coping and distress, personality, substance abuse, and other present and past psychiatric disorders (e.g., major depression, anxiety disorder, or severe personality disorder), can be exceedingly complex and require assessment by a specialist.

The experience of pain often has a profound effect on the patient's family and others in the social milieu. The issues are again complex. Some families provide essential support and cope well. Others may disintegrate under the pressure of dealing with the patient's chronic pain. Caregiver burden is an underrecognized concern in the management of chronic pain. Still other families appear to become part of the problem of disability. Chronic pain can be used as an interpersonal device by some patients, and families may erect pain-reinforcing behavioral contingencies (such as strong encouragement to reduce function) without insight into the adverse consequences of doing so. Through family meetings, individual clinicians can directly address some of these contingencies as part of the treatment plan.

Assessing Other Relevant History

The pain assessment also may benefit from several other details. The reactions of the patient and family to prior diseases may be informative, particularly if this history includes periods of protracted illness. For example, a history of illness associated with vocational changes, lifestyle changes, increased dependency on family members and health care resources, and other evidence of functional decline may suggest more aggressive rehabilitative interventions earlier in the course of painful illness.

A specific history of painful disorders, including recurrent back pain, dysmenorrhea, abdominal pain, and headaches, is similarly important. Information about the nature and outcome of the physical and psychosocial comorbidities that may have been associated with these pains can provide valuable insights into the current pain problem.

As noted, a history of drug use is a particularly important dimension of the pain assessment. This history should address the use of all types of drugs, including alcohol, prescription drugs, over-the-counter remedies, and both licit and illicit drugs (Passik and Portenoy 1998; Portenoy and Payne 1997).

Conclusion

Pain is an extremely prevalent and heterogeneous symptom that often challenges clinicians and profoundly distresses patients. Persistent pain is best approached clinically from the perspective of a biopsychosocial model, which acknowledges that pain and pain-related disability arise through the complex interplay of nociceptive and nonnociceptive factors. These nonnociceptive factors are often psychological or psychosocial.

Much of the data necessary to develop a differential diagnosis for the pain and to formulate a pain-oriented problem list can be gleaned from a careful history. Dimensions of the pain experience that should be explored include temporal features, pain distribution, pain intensity, pain quality, and exacerbating and alleviating factors. The history should clarify psychiatric comorbidity, including the use of licit and illicit drugs. The response to prior pain experiences and coping strategies used during times of stress may provide important guidance in the formulation of an effective treatment plan.

Combined with a physical examination and appropriate laboratory and imaging studies, this history can identify the pain syndrome, clarify the etiology and pathophysiology of the pain, and guide the selection of therapeutic interventions. As the therapeutic arsenal available to treat pain expands, it becomes even more important to comprehensively evaluate patients with chronic pain. In this way, treatment can be optimized, and patients may be spared the expense, risk, and inconvenience of inappropriate therapies.

References

American Psychiatric Association: Diagnostic and Statistical Manual of Mental Disorders, 4th Edition. Washington, DC, American Psychiatric Association, 1994

Arner S, Myerson BA: Lack of analgesic effect of opioids on neuropathic and idiopathic forms of pain. Pain 33:11–23, 1988

Au E, Loprinzi CL, Dhodapkar M, et al: Regular use of verbal pain scale improves the understanding of oncology inpatient pain intensity. J Clin Oncol 12:2751–2755, 1994

Banos JE, Bosch F, Canellas M, et al: Acceptability of visual analogue scales in the clinical setting: a comparison with verbal rating scales in postoperative pain. Methods Find Exp Clin Pharmacol 11:123–127, 1989

Besson J-M, Chaouch A: Peripheral and spinal mechanisms of nociception. Physiol Rev 67:67–185, 1987

Bonica JJ: Definitions and taxonomy of pain, in The Management of Pain. Edited by Bonica JJ. Philadelphia, PA, Lea & Febiger, 1990, pp 18–27

Chapman CR, Casey KL, Dubner R, et al: Pain measurement: an overview. Pain 22:1–31, 1985

Cousins M: Acute and postoperative pain, in Textbook of Pain, 3rd Edition. Edited by Wall PD, Melzack R. Edinburgh, Churchill Livingstone, 1994, pp 357–387

Daut RL, Cleeland CS, Flanery RC: Development of the Wisconsin Brief Pain Questionnaire to assess pain in cancer and other diseases. Pain 17:197–210, 1983

De Conno F, Caraceni A, Gamba A, et al: Pain measurement in cancer patients: a comparison of six methods. Pain 57:161–166, 1994

Edwards WT: Optimizing opioid treatment of postoperative pain. J Pain Symptom Manage 5:S24–S36, 1990

Engel GL: The need for a new medical model: a challenge for biomedicine. Science 196(4286):129–136, 1977

Foley KM: The treatment of cancer pain. N Engl J Med 313:84–95, 1985

Gonzales GR, Elliott KJ, Portenoy RK, et al: The impact of a comprehensive evaluation in the management of cancer pain. Pain 47:141–144, 1991

Gracely RH, Kwilosz DM: The Descriptor Differential Scale: applying psychophysical principles to clinical pain assessment. Pain 35:279–288, 1988

Health and Public Policy Committee, American College of Physicians: Drug therapy for severe chronic pain in terminal illness. Ann Intern Med 99:870–873, 1983

Jacox A, Carr DB, Payne R, et al: Management of cancer pain: Clinical Practice Guideline No 9 (AHCPR Publ No 94-0592). Rockville, MD, U.S. Department of Health and Human Services, Public Health Service, 1994

Jensen MP, McFarland CA: Increasing the reliability and validity of pain intensity measurement in chronic pain patients. Pain 55:195–203, 1993

Kerns RD, Turk DC, Rudy TE: The West Haven–Yale Multidimensional Pain Inventory (WHYMPI). Pain 23:345–356, 1985

Loeser JD, Egan KJ: History and organization of the University of Washington Multidisciplinary Pain Center, in Managing the Chronic Pain Patient: Theory and Practice at the University of Washington Multidisciplinary Pain Center. Edited by Loeser JD, Egan, KJ. New York, Raven, 1989, pp 3–20

Margoles MS: The pain chart: spatial properties of pain, in Pain Measurement and Assessment. Edited by Melzack R. New York, Raven, 1983, pp 215–231

McGivney WT, Crooks GM: The care of patients with severe chronic pain in terminal illness. JAMA 251:1182–1188, 1984

Melzack R: The McGill Pain Questionnaire: major properties and scoring methods. Pain 1:277–299, 1975

Melzack R, Casey KL: Sensory, motivational, and central control determinants of pain: a new conceptual model, in The Skin Senses. Edited by Kenshalo D. Springfield, IL, Charles C Thomas, 1968, pp 423–429

Merskey H, Bogduk N: Classification of Chronic Pain, 2nd Edition. Seattle, WA, IASP Press, 1994

Passik SD, Portenoy RK: Substance abuse issues in psycho-oncology, in Psycho-Oncology. Edited by Holland JH, Breitbart W, Jacobsen P, et al. Oxford, England, Oxford University Press, 1998, pp 576–586

Perry S, Heidrich G: Management of pain during debridement: a survey of U.S. burn units. Pain 13:267–280, 1982

Portenoy RK: Contemporary Diagnosis and Management of Pain in Oncologic and AIDS Patients. Newtown, PA, Handbooks in Health Care, 1997

Portenoy RK, Cheville AL: Chronic pain management, in Psychiatric Care of the Medical Patient, 2nd Edition. Edited by Stoudemire A, Fogel BS, Greenberg DB. New York, Oxford University Press, 2000, pp 199–225

Portenoy RK, Foley KM: Chronic use of opioid analgesics in non-malignant pain: report of 38 cases. Pain 25:171–186, 1986

Portenoy RK, Foley KM: The management of cancer pain, in Handbook of Psycho-Oncology: Psychological Care of the Patient With Cancer. Edited by Holland JC, Roland JH. New York, Oxford University Press, 1989, pp 369–382

Portenoy RK, Hagen NA: Breakthrough pain: definition, prevalence and characteristics. Pain 41:273–281, 1990

Portenoy RK, Payne R: Acute and chronic pain, in Comprehensive Textbook of Substance Abuse, 3rd Edition. Edited by Lowinson JH, Ruiz P, Millman RB. Baltimore, MD, Williams & Wilkins, 1997, pp 563–590

Portenoy RK, Foley KM, Inturrisi CE: The nature of opioid responsiveness and its implications for neuropathic pain: new hypotheses derived from studies of opioid infusions. Pain 43:273–286, 1990

Portenoy RK, Payne DK, Jacobsen P: Breakthrough pain: characteristics and impact in patients with cancer pain. Pain 81:129–134, 1999

Price DD: Psychological and Neural Mechanisms of Pain. New York, Raven, 1988, pp 28–38

Romano JM, Turner JA: Chronic pain and depression: does the evidence support a relationship? Psychol Bull 97:18–34, 1985

Swerdlow M, Stjernsward J: Cancer pain relief—an urgent problem. World Health Forum 3:325–330, 1982

Torebjork HE, Ochoa JL, Schary W: Referred pain from intraneural stimulation of muscle fascicles in the median nerve. Pain 118:145–156, 1984

Turk DC, Rudy TE: The robustness of an empirically derived taxonomy of chronic pain patients. Pain 43:27–35, 1990

Turk DC, Rudy TE: Toward an empirically derived taxonomy of chronic pain patients: integration of psychological assessment data. J Consult Clin Psychol 56:233–238, 1988

Wirth FP, Van Buren JM: Referral of pain from dural stimulation in man. J Neurosurg 34:630–642, 1971

World Health Organization: Cancer Pain Relief, 2nd Edition, With a Guide to Opioid Availability. Geneva, World Health Organization, 1996

Yaksh TL: An introductory perspective on the study of nociception and its modulation, in Anesthesia: Biologic Foundations. Edited by Yaksh TL, Lynch C, Zapol W, et al. Philadelphia, PA, JB Lippincott, 1998, pp 471–483

Chapter 2

Pain Management

Pharmacological and Nonpharmacological Treatments

Augusto Caraceni, M.D.
Andrea Cheville, M.D.
Russell K. Portenoy, M.D.

The management of chronic pain is predicated on a comprehensive assessment of the pain itself, coexisting physical and psychosocial disabilities, and other comorbid conditions. This assessment can guide a therapeutic strategy that may involve the combined use of multiple modalities targeted to the pain or related problems. The very large number of treatment modalities used specifically for pain can be broadly categorized as pharmacological, anesthesiological, surgical, neurostimulatory, physiatric, psychological, and complementary.

Chronic pain is extraordinarily heterogeneous, and the decision to use one or more therapeutic modalities as well as the emphasis that each approach receives in a multimodality strategy must be individualized. For some patients, pharmacotherapy should be the sole approach, or at least strongly emphasized. For others, the use of analgesic drugs is appropriately minimized, and the strategy should focus on other treatments, such as physical or cognitive therapy. A subpopulation of patients with chronic nonmalignant pain associated with disturbances in diverse areas of function may be best managed by referral to a multidisciplinary pain management program.

Because of this complexity, all clinicians involved in the care of patients with chronic pain should have a broad understanding of the range of therapeutic options now available. The following sections offer a detailed review of analgesic pharmacotherapy and some of the more useful nonpharmacological interventions.

Nonopioid Analgesics

Nonsteroidal anti-inflammatory drugs (NSAIDs) and acetaminophen, the most widely used first-line analgesics for acute and chronic pain, comprise an extremely diverse group of drugs (Table 2–1). The analgesic activity of NSAIDs is mediated by the inhibition of the enzyme cyclooxygenase (COX), which reduces the synthesis of prostaglandins. Prostaglandins are key inflammatory mediators and sensitize primary afferent nerves that respond to noxious stimuli in the periphery.

Although inhibition of these peripheral processes can explain both the analgesic and the anti-inflammatory effects of the NSAIDs, prostaglandin inhibition in the central nervous system (CNS) also probably contributes to the analgesic effects (Willer et al. 1989). The central effects of the NSAIDs presumably account for their antipyretic activity and for the observed disparity between the anti-inflammatory and analgesic potencies of some of these drugs (McCormack and Brune 1991).

The enzyme COX exists in at least two physiological forms: COX-1 (constitutive) and COX-2 (inducible). Most NSAIDs are nonspecific inhibitors of both isoforms. The inhibition of COX-1 is associated with the renal and gastric toxicities of these drugs, whereas the inhibition of COX-2 reduces inflammation and is presumably more responsible for the therapeutic effects. COX-2–selective inhibitors, specifically celecoxib and rofecoxib, are now commercially available in the United States, and another NSAID that is available in Europe, nimesulide, has a prevailing COX-2–inhibiting effect. These drugs have less gastrointestinal (GI) toxicity than the nonselective COX inhibitors and will likely play an expanding role in analgesic therapy.

Acetaminophen is only marginally effective in the peripheral synthesis of prostaglandins. It reduces prostaglandin production in the CNS, and this mechanism presumably underlies both the analgesic and the antipyretic effects of this drug. Although acetaminophen is often regarded as having a less potent analgesic effect than full-dose NSAID therapy, it is nonetheless a useful analgesic (McQuay and Moore 1998).

Table 2–1. Nonsteroidal anti-inflammatory drugs (NSAIDs)

Group and drug	Total daily dose (mg)[a]	Dosing interval	Half-life (hours)
Salicylates			
Choline magnesium trisalicylate	1,500–4,000	q12h	9–17
Salsalate	3,000	q12h	16
Diflunisal	1,000–1,500	q12h	8–12
Indoles			
Indomethacin	50–150	q8h–q6h	4.5
Sulindac	200–400	q12h	8
Tolmetin	600–1,800	q8h	2–5
Etodolac	600–1,600	q4h–q6h	3–11
Propionic acids			
Ibuprofen	1,200–3,200	q4h–q6h	2
Flurbiprofen	100–300	q12h	5.7
Fenoprofen	900–2,400	q8h–q6h	3
Ketoprofen	150–300	q8h–q6h	2–4
Naproxen	275–1,375	q12h	13
Fenamates[b]			
Mefenamic acid	1,000	q6h	2
Meclofenamate	200–600	q4h–q6h	2
Others			
Piroxicam	20–40	qd	50
Nabumetone	1,000–2,000	qd–q12h	24
Ketorolac	10–40	q6h	4–7
Diclofenac	100–150	q8h–q6h	2
Selective cyclooxygenase-2 inhibitors[c]			
Celecoxib	200–400	q12h	—
Rofecoxib	12.5–25	q24h	—

[a]Initial and full maximum daily doses are given.
[b]These drugs are not recommended for prolonged use because of increased risk of gastrointestinal toxicity. Metabolites are active, and their half-lives are long enough to allow less frequent dosing.
[c]All the other NSAIDs are nonselective cyclooxygenase-1 and cyclooxygenase-2 inhibitors.
Source. Adapted from Caraceni and Portenoy (in press).

Drug Selection

Both NSAIDs and acetaminophen have dose-dependent effects and a ceiling effect for analgesia. The existence of ceiling doses implies that these drugs have limited maximal efficacy. As a result, they are typically considered for patients with pain that is generally mild or moderate.

Each NSAID has large individual variation in the minimal effective dose, toxic dose, and ceiling dose. Dose titration is often needed to identify the optimal dose for an individual patient. There is also very large individual variation in the analgesic response to different drugs in this category. This observation suggests that patients who are candidates for treatment with a nonopioid drug often benefit from sequential trials if outcomes are not favorable initially.

Another source of variability in the individual response to NSAIDs and acetaminophen is the type of pain. NSAIDs appear to be particularly effective in pain related to grossly inflammatory processes or injury to bone. They seem to be relatively less useful for neuropathic pain. These observations have never been systematically confirmed, however, and it is most appropriate at this time to consider these drugs as nonspecific analgesics that potentially could be useful for any type of chronic pain.

Acetaminophen is safer than any of the currently available NSAIDs and is, therefore, often considered first if a nonopioid is desired for mild pain. It is also often considered as a coanalgesic if another type of drug is the focus of therapy. Both NSAIDs and acetaminophen enhance opioid analgesia and reduce the opioid dose required (McQuay and Moore 1998; Mercadante et al. 1997).

Drug Toxicities

The potential for serious toxicity should influence the decision to initiate analgesic therapy. High doses of acetaminophen can produce severe hepatic injury. In patients with no preexisting liver disease, long-term administration of 4 g/day or less is typically considered safe. Patients with significant liver disease and those with a history of heavy alcohol use are predisposed to this toxicity and should be limited to lower doses. Cirrhosis should be considered a strong relative contraindication to this drug.

GI symptoms occur in about 10% of the patients treated with

traditional NSAIDs (nonselective COX inhibitors), and ulcers occur in about 2% (Loeb et al. 1992). Although some surveys suggest that the risk is limited to gastric ulceration, other data implicate both gastric and duodenal lesions.

Importantly, GI symptoms are poor predictors of serious GI toxicity. Two-thirds of NSAID-related GI hemorrhages or perforations occur without preceding GI symptoms. As a result, clinicians cannot wait until symptoms of toxicity occur to decide whether to continue therapy, reduce the dose, or switch to a safer regimen. The risks must be assessed before therapy, and appropriate measures taken before adverse events occur.

An increased risk of ulceration is associated with advanced age, the use of higher doses of NSAIDs, concomitant administration of a corticosteroid, and a history of either ulcer disease or previous GI complications from NSAIDs (Loeb et al. 1992; Simon 1993). Heavy alcohol or cigarette consumption also may increase the risk. Although infection with *Helicobacter pylori* may have a role in NSAID-related gastropathy, this has not yet been proven (Schubert et al. 1993).

The potential for GI toxicity differs substantially among the various NSAIDs, but comparative epidemiological data are limited (Langman et al. 1994). Many drugs have not been adequately evaluated, and the relative risk can be inferred only from the rates of adverse events recorded during drug development and postmarketing surveys. The existing data suggest that the long-term GI toxicity profiles are relatively favorable for some drugs, such as ibuprofen, choline magnesium trisalicylate, ketoprofen, diclofenac, nabumetone, and oxaprozin, and relatively unfavorable for others, such as aspirin, piroxicam, and ketorolac.

A relatively high risk of GI toxicity suggests the use of a COX-2–selective drug or a concomitant gastroprotective therapy. Gastroprotection can be achieved with misoprostol, a prostaglandin analogue that reduces the incidence of NSAID-induced ulcers; a proton pump inhibitor, such as omeprazole; or higher-dose histamine H_2 blocker therapy (Numo 1992; Taha et al. 1996; M. N. Wolfe et al. 1999). Other interventions, such as antacids and sucralfate, may reduce symptoms but have never been shown to decrease the risk of NSAID-induced ulceration.

NSAIDs can cause serious renal toxicity (Murray and Brater 1993). They should not be used in patients who have clinically evident renal disease and should be used with caution in patients who are likely to have subclinical disease as a result of advanced age, dehydration, prior treatment with nephrotoxic therapy (such as aminoglycosides or platinum-based chemotherapy), or an underlying disease. Although there is a theoretical reason to believe that the COX-2–selective NSAIDs will be associated with less renal toxicity and will be substantially safer for patients with renal disease than the nonselective COX inhibitors, no empirical support for this theory exists.

NSAID-induced inhibition of platelet aggregation is a serious concern in some patients, such as those with a preexisting coagulopathy and those who are medically frail and could not tolerate an episode of bleeding. The antiplatelet effect of a single dose of aspirin is irreversible and can double the bleeding time for up to 1 week. Other NSAIDs have reversible effects on platelet function and affect bleeding time only while circulating in the plasma. Acetaminophen does not inhibit platelet function and is preferred if the risk of bleeding is high. Although the nonacetylated salicylates, such as choline magnesium trisalicylate and salsalate, have minimal effects on platelets and should theoretically pose less risk, the safety of these drugs in patients predisposed to bleeding has not been established in the clinical setting. Similarly, the effects of the COX-2–selective drugs on platelets should be relatively less than those of nonselective COX inhibitors, but this has not been established in clinical studies.

Some patients develop other types of adverse effects from NSAID therapy. CNS effects, such as dizziness, confusion, or headache, can occur (and are relatively more common with some drugs such as indomethacin). Hypersensitivity reactions vary from very mild cutaneous eruptions to life-threatening anaphylaxis. If a patient develops allergy, cross-reactivity across all the NSAIDs, including aspirin, should be assumed.

Dosing and Monitoring

Numerous NSAIDs are available (Table 2–1), and most are available in a range of doses. This permits the use of dose titration when initiating treatment. It is reasonable to begin therapy at a relatively low dose when patients report mild to moderate pain or are at a relatively increased risk for NSAID toxicity, such as occurs in the elderly. In the absence of factors that increase the risk of therapy, higher or full starting doses can be used in patients with more acute or severe pain. The only NSAID available for parenteral use in the United States, ketorolac, is recommended for short-term use in patients with acute pain and is usually administered with a loading dose (usually 30 mg).

Patients who do not experience adequate analgesia within a week of starting therapy can be considered for dose escalation. Dose escalation is limited by the occurrence of a ceiling effect (indicated by the failure to obtain additional analgesia after the dose is increased), by concerns about increased risk, and by conventional practice. The conventional maximal dose of most drugs is one to two times the starting dose. If the maximal dose is reached without achieving satisfactory analgesia, an alternative NSAID trial can be considered.

The monitoring of patients receiving NSAID therapy should be individualized. This monitoring might include a test for occult fecal blood and an evaluation of hemoglobin and renal and hepatic function. Patients who develop severe GI symptoms may be considered for upper GI endoscopy. Patients who are predisposed to adverse effects and those who are receiving relatively high doses should be monitored more frequently.

Adjuvant Analgesics

The term *adjuvant analgesic* is used to describe a drug that has a primary indication other than pain but may be analgesic in specific circumstances (Portenoy 1990). This definition evolved in a literature that described the use of these drugs in combination with traditional analgesics, specifically opioids. The utility of many of these agents has steadily expanded, and they now have a clear role as primary analgesics for many types of pain. Although the description of such drugs as adjuvants is a misnomer, it continues nonetheless and does suggest the potential utility of analgesic drug combinations, particularly those that link drugs of varied mechanisms (Brose and Cousins 1991; Caraceni et al. 1999; Mercadante et al. 1998; Sandford et al. 1992; Tanelian and Cousins 1989).

Antidepressants

As shown in a recent systematic review (McQuay and Moore 1998), tricyclic antidepressants (TCAs) are analgesic in numerous chronic pain states (Bowsher 1997; Butler 1984; Getto et al. 1987; Goldenberg et al. 1996; Max et al. 1991; Kani et al. 1996). Analgesic effects are not dependent on an antidepressant effect, as initially postulated (Evans et al. 1973). Analgesia typically occurs earlier than mood change in chronic pain patients and can occur in both nondepressed chronic pain patients and depressed patients who do not have a favorable mood change during treatment (Couch et al. 1976; Kishore-Kumar et al. 1990; Max et al. 1987; Watson et al. 1982). Analgesic effects also have been shown in animal models (Spiegel et al. 1983).

The analgesic action of TCAs is probably related to their ability to inhibit the reuptake of serotonin and norepinephrine at the synaptic cleft. This activity may inhibit nociceptive transmission at the first central synapse in the dorsal horn of the spinal cord by facilitating the descending inhibitory serotonergic and noradrenergic tracts that originate in the rostroventral medulla (Besson and Chaouch 1987; Hammond 1985; Yaksh 1998). The tertiary amine TCA drugs (e.g., amitriptyline) exert their greatest effect on serotonin, and the secondary amine TCA drugs (e.g., desipramine) have relatively greater effects on norepinephrine.

Numerous controlled trials have established the analgesic efficacy of specific TCAs. Amitriptyline, for example, has been shown to relieve pain in patients with diabetic neuropathy (Max et al. 1987; Vrethem et al. 1997); postherpetic neuralgia (Watson et al. 1982); tension and migraine headache (Cerbo et al. 1998; Couch et al. 1976); genital, pelvic, and suprapubic pain syndromes (Pranikoff and Constantino 1998); fibromyalgia (Goldenberg et al. 1996); nerve injury following breast cancer treatment (Kalso et al. 1996); and psychogenic pain (Pilowsky et al. 1982). A recent randomized, controlled trial found that preemptive administration of low-dose amitriptyline reduced pain prevalence in patients with herpes zoster (Bowsher 1997). Imipramine has been found to be effective in patients with arthritic pain (Gingras 1976) and painful diabetic neuropathy (Kvinsdahl et al. 1984), and doxepin has been found to be effective in patients with psychogenic headache (Okasha et al. 1973) or concurrent chronic pain and depression (Hameroff et al. 1982). Clomipramine has had analgesic effects in several pain syndromes (Langohr et al. 1982), and desipramine has been effective in patients with postherpetic neuralgia (Kishore-Kumar et al. 1990) and diabetic neuropathy (Max et al. 1991).

Much less information about the newer antidepressants, including the selective serotonin reuptake inhibitors (SSRIs), is available. Fluoxetine has been anecdotally reported to benefit both phantom limb pain (Power-Smith and Turkington 1993) and pain secondary to diabetic neuropathy (Theesan and Marsh 1989). Results of controlled trials of fluoxetine in patients with fibromyalgia were equivocal (Goldenberg et al. 1996; F. Wolfe et al. 1994), and in other controlled trials, fluoxetine offered no benefit over placebo in the management of painful diabetic neuropathy (Max et al. 1992) and yielded slightly reduced frequency but no change in intensity of headache (Saper et al. 1994). Paroxetine provided significant pain relief at a dose range of 30–70 mg/day in a controlled comparison against imipramine in patients with diabetic neuropathy (Sindrup et al. 1990). The use of lower doses, specifically 20–30 mg/day, may account for the negative findings in a later study of paroxetine for prophylaxis of chronic tension-type headache (Langemark and Olesen 1994). Although other trials were not favorable, a controlled study of citalopram in painful diabetic neuropathy yielded positive results (Sindrup et al. 1992).

Trazodone, which also has a prevailing serotonergic effect, seemed effective in one study of patients with cancer-related neuropathic pain (Ventafridda et al. 1987a) but could not be separated from placebo when tested in patients with painful traumatic myelopathy (Davidoff et al. 1987) or chronic low back pain (Goodkin et al. 1990). Another serotonergic drug, zimelidine, had an analgesic effect in a controlled trial of patients with mixed organic and psychogenic pain syndromes (Johansson and Von Knorring 1979) but was ineffective in an open-label comparison with amitriptyline in patients with postherpetic neuralgia (Watson and Evans 1985). The noradrenergic drug maprotiline was favorably compared with clomipramine in idiopathic pain (Eberhard et al. 1988) and amitriptyline in postherpetic neuralgia (Watson et al. 1990) and painful polyneuropathy (Vrethem et al. 1997).

Monoamine oxidase inhibitors (MAOIs) increase the availability of central monoamines, and sparse data suggest analgesic effects from these compounds as well. Their analgesic potential was suggested by one open-label study of refractory migraine (Anthony and Lance 1969) and a controlled trial of patients with atypical facial pain (Lascelles 1966). Their potential for toxicity, however—specifically, hypertensive crisis after the ingestion of tyramine-containing foods and numerous drugs—limits their utility. They are now generally used only for refractory migraine headache. If an MAOI is used, patient education regarding dietary restrictions and drugs to avoid is mandatory. For patients with pain, the potential interaction of an MAOI with meperidine should be particularly emphasized; this combination can produce a life-threatening hyperpyrexic syndrome.

Given the broad range of pain syndromes that have responded favorably in studies, the antidepressants should be considered nonspecific analgesics. These drugs may be considered for most chronic pain syndromes. The justification for a trial is particularly strong if the patient has a comorbid depression or an associated sleep disturbance.

Because of their anticholinergic effects, TCAs are relatively contraindicated for patients with significant cardiac arrhythmias, symptomatic prostatic hypertrophy, narrow angle glaucoma, and other relevant medical conditions. Although tertiary amine TCAs, particularly amitriptyline, are often considered first for pain because of the extensive supporting evidence, these drugs have a more troublesome side-effect profile than the secondary amine TCAs. Accordingly, patients who cannot tolerate the sedative, anticholinergic, or hypotensive effects of amitriptyline or another tertiary amine TCA should be considered for a trial with a secondary amine TCA. Desipramine has been the most carefully studied, and there is good support for its analgesic efficacy.

Patients who are unlikely to tolerate a TCA, or who have had intolerable side effects from a secondary amine drug, are often considered for a trial of a newer antidepressant. As noted, some evidence from controlled trials supports the analgesic effects of drugs such as paroxetine, citalopram, fluoxetine, and maprotiline, and anecdotal reports have suggested that others, such as venlafaxine and nefazodone, can be helpful. At this time, the selection of these drugs for patients with chronic pain is guided mostly by clinical experience.

When TCAs are administered for pain, they generally should be started at a low dose, such as 10–25 mg at night. Doses are gradually increased over several weeks. Analgesic effects usually occur within 4–7 days after an effective dose is reached, and for all the aforementioned TCAs, the effective dose is usually in the range of 50–150 mg/day (Kishore-Kumar et al. 1990; Max et al. 1987; Watson et al. 1982). Studies have suggested that analgesia is a dose-dependent effect (Max et al. 1987), and upward titration of the dose should be continued if neither analgesia nor intolerable side effects occur in the usual therapeutic range. Higher doses also may be needed if a coexistent depression is prominent. A single nighttime dose is adequate for most patients, but analgesic effects wane toward evening in some patients, who would benefit more from twice-daily dosing. Plasma level monitoring can be used to determine the lack of compliance, poor absorption, or unusually rapid catabolism. Analgesic plasma levels are unknown.

α_2-*Adrenergic Agonists*

Clonidine and tizanidine inhibit central adrenergic transmission as a result of their agonist action on the α_2-adrenergic receptors. These drugs have established analgesic effects in a variety of pain syndromes (headache, diabetic neuropathy pain, postoperative pain, postherpetic neuralgia, and cancer pain) (Byas-Smith et al. 1995; Hirata et al. 1995). Thus, these adjuvant analgesics, like the antidepressants, are appropriately considered nonspecific analgesics. A study of transdermal clonidine administration in patients with postherpetic neuralgia supported the potential for analgesia but found that a relatively small proportion of patients respond (Byas-Smith et al. 1995).

Clonidine administration can cause hypotension, which may

limit its usefulness as an analgesic. Among those without serious medical illness, however, somnolence and dry mouth are the more frequent side effects. Given the relatively poor response rate and the potential for toxicity, this drug usually is considered only after several other adjuvant analgesics have failed. If a trial is undertaken, either the oral or the transdermal route can be used. Treatment should begin with a very low dose (e.g., 0.05–0.1 mg/day). Clonidine also has been administered via the spinal route in patients with cancer pain (see "Intraspinal Drug Administration," later in this chapter).

Tizanidine, which is commercially marketed in the United States for the indication of spasticity, is also a nonspecific analgesic. Somnolence is the most difficult side effect, and hypotension is less common than with clonidine. Like clonidine, tizanidine treatment should be started with a low dose (2–4 mg) that is gradually increased if tolerated.

Corticosteroids

The corticosteroids have been shown to be useful in the supportive care of patients with advanced medical illness by improving pain, appetite, nausea, malaise, and overall quality of life (Bruera et al. 1985; Della Cuna et al. 1989; Tannock et al. 1989). Several pain-related indications are well accepted in the cancer population, including neuropathic pain, bone pain, pain associated with hepatic capsular expansion or duct obstruction, pain due to bowel obstruction, pain caused by lymphedema, pain due to epidural spinal cord compression, and headache due to increased intracranial pressure. In patients with advanced disease, the risk-benefit ratio has been considered sufficiently favorable to justify long-term therapy, typically with low doses. In a large survey of patients with advanced cancer, the most common adverse effect during prolonged treatment was oral candidiasis (Hanks et al. 1983).

In populations with nonmalignant pain, corticosteroids also may be considered nonspecific analgesics, but the potential for long-term toxicity limits the use of these drugs to short-term therapy for specific indications (such as complex regional pain syndrome [also known as reflex sympathetic dystrophy and causalgia], acute radiculopathy, and severe vascular headache) and to long-term therapy for pain associated with inflammatory diseases (such as rheumatoid arthritis or inflammatory bowel syndrome). The serious adverse effects of these drugs include an increased risk of infection, myopathy, diabetes, fluid overload (ranging from peripheral edema to congestive heart failure), cushingoid habitus, increased risk of skin breakdown, GI perforation, and neuropsychiatric syndromes (ranging from mild dysphoria or mental clouding to severe anxiety or depression, or even psychosis).

There is no evidence that the available corticosteroid drugs vary in analgesic efficacy. If mineralocorticoid effects are a concern, dexamethasone is preferred. The typical approach to dosing involves treatment with the lowest effective dose. In the cancer population, a high-dose regimen (e.g., dexamethasone 100 mg followed by 24 mg every 6 hours and a rapid taper thereafter) is used for crescendo pain and selected oncological emergencies (most notably, acute spinal cord compression).

Anticonvulsants

Any of the aforementioned nonspecific adjuvant analgesics may be used to treat neuropathic pain. In addition, many drugs are used selectively for this type of pain. In most cases, this reflects clinical experience and the range of pain syndromes addressed in clinical trials. Future studies may indicate that some of these drugs, or drug classes, are as nonspecific in their potential to yield analgesia as the antidepressants. Efforts have been made to provide evidence-based guidelines for the selection of drugs for neuropathic pain (McQuay and Moore 1998), but the number and range of controlled clinical trials are limited, and clinicians are well served by being familiar with the broad array of drugs that are now used by pain specialists.

The role of anticonvulsant drugs as analgesics for neuropathic pain is evolving. Currently, gabapentin often is considered a first-line drug for neuropathic pain of any type. The other drugs in this class usually are selected early when the pain syndrome is characterized by a lancinating or paroxysmal component (McQuay and Moore 1998; Swerdlow 1984). Clinical experience suggests, however, that any of these drugs potentially can be useful even when the neuropathic pain lacks a paroxysmal component (Max et al. 1992).

The modes of analgesic action for these drugs probably vary (Table 2–2). Analgesia could relate to inhibition of membrane sodium channels in some cases or to modulation of the inhibitory neurotransmitter γ-aminobutyric acid (GABA) in others (Rall and Schleifer 1985). Anticonvulsants presumably attenuate the ectopic electrical activity in peripheral or central neural structures that has been implicated in the generation of dysesthetic pain (Albe-Fessard and Lombard 1982; Loeser et al. 1968; Nystrom and Hagbarth 1981; Wall and Gutnick 1974). Anticonvulsant blockade of aberrant sodium channel activity has been seen in nociceptive neurons (Devor 1994).

Gabapentin is the anticonvulsant that is now most widely administered for pain. It is commonly used for neuropathic pain of any type and for migraine prophylaxis. The analgesic efficacy of this drug is supported by controlled clinical trials in postherpetic neuralgia and painful diabetic neuropathy (Backonja et al. 1998; Rowbotham et al. 1998) and by anecdotal reports in patients with neuropathic head and neck pain, postherpetic neuralgia, dysesthetic limb pain in multiple sclerosis, trigeminal neuralgia, erythromelalgia, sympathetically maintained pain, and radiation myelopathy (Caraceni et al. 1999; McGraw and Koseck 1997; Mellick and Mellick 1997; Rosenberg et al. 1997; Samkoff et al. 1997; Segal and Rordorf 1996; Sist et al. 1997a, 1997b).

Gabapentin has an unknown mechanism of action. The possibilities include inhibition of glutamate synthesis, binding to a novel calcium channel, or enhancement of the releasable pool of GABA in the CNS (Gee et al. 1996; Goldlust et al. 1995; Koesis and Honmou 1994). Experimental data suggest a specific antihyperalgesic activity for gabapentin and related compounds (Field et al. 1997).

A relatively low starting dose, such as 300 mg/day (even lower in the elderly and medically frail patients), of gabapentin is typically used. Dose escalation over a period of days is usually required to reach the effective analgesic dose, which is in the range of 900–3,600 mg/day and sometimes higher. The drug is not me-

Table 2–2. Anticonvulsants used for pain management and their relevant principles of action

Drug	Decrease in sodium channel activity	Increase in CNS GABA activity	Modulation of Ca^{2+} channels	Reduction of excitatory amino acid activity
Carbamazepine	+			
Phenytoin	+			
Valproate	+	+	+	
Gabapentin	+	+	+ (?)	
Lamotrigine	+			
Felbamate		+		+
Topiramate	+	+		+
Vigabatrin		+		
Tiagabine		+		

Note. CNS = central nervous system; GABA = γ-aminobutyric acid; Ca^{2+} = calcium.

tabolized by the liver and has no pharmacokinetic interactions with other drugs. Therefore, the risk of serious toxicity is low. However, side effects, including somnolence, mental clouding, mood changes, and lower limb edema, are common.

Phenytoin was the first anticonvulsant used to treat neuropathic pain. Initial case reports suggested efficacy in trigeminal neuralgia (Blom 1963; Braham and Saia 1960), and favorable effects were reported in patients with glossopharyngeal neuralgia, tabetic lightning pains, paroxysmal pain in postherpetic neuralgia, thalamic pain, postsympathectomy pain, and posttraumatic neuralgia (Cantor 1972; Green 1961; Hatangdi et al. 1976; Raskin et al. 1974; Swerdlow and Cundill 1981; Taylor et al. 1977). Controlled trials in patients with painful neuropathy from Fabry's disease (Lockman et al. 1973) and painful diabetic neuropathy (Chadda and Mathur 1978) had similar outcomes.

Carbamazepine has established efficacy in trigeminal neuralgia (Campbell et al. 1966; Killian and Fromm 1968; Rockliff and Davis 1966), in the lancinating (but not continuous) pains of postherpetic neuralgia (Killian and Fromm 1968), and in painful diabetic neuropathy (Rull et al. 1969). Published case series and anecdotal reports also have suggested benefit in glossopharyngeal neuralgia, tabetic lightning pains, paroxysmal pain in multiple sclerosis, postsympathectomy pain, lancinating pains due to cancer, and posttraumatic neuralgia (Ekbom 1972; Elliot et al. 1976; Espir and Millac 1970; Mullan 1973; Raskin et al. 1974; Swerdlow and Cundill 1981; Tanelian and Cousins 1989; Taylor et al. 1977).

Uncontrolled clinical trials and anecdotal reports have similarly suggested that clonazepam and valproate may be effective in neuropathic pain characterized by lancinating dysesthesias (Caccia 1975; Martin 1981; Peiris et al. 1980; Raftery 1979; Swerdlow and Cundill 1981). However, valproate was found to be equal to placebo in the treatment of chronic central dysesthetic pain following spinal cord injury (Drewes et al. 1994). Valproate has established activity as a prophylactic agent for migraine headache (Jensen et al. 1994; Rothrock 1997; Silberstein 1996).

Lamotrigine was effective in controlled trials that evaluated patients with refractory trigeminal neuralgia (Zakrzewska et al. 1997) and patients with pain following transurethral prostatectomy (Bonicalzi et al. 1997). In contrast, lamotrigine showed no benefit over placebo in the prophylaxis of migraine headache (Steiner et al. 1997). This drug has a relatively high risk of cutaneous hypersensitivity reactions, including the serious adverse outcome of Stevens-Johnson syndrome. To reduce this risk, dosing must start at only 25–50 mg/day, then increase slowly over 1 month. The drug is not indicated for children younger than 15 years, who are at increased risk for rash.

An anecdotal report noted that felbamate was analgesic in refractory trigeminal neuralgia (Cheshire 1995). Interest in the use of the drug as an analgesic waned, however, when it became associated with life-threatening aplastic anemia.

Other new anticonvulsants, including tiagabine and topiramate, have not yet been evaluated as analgesics. Clinical observations suggest that both could potentially benefit selected patients with neuropathic pain, but clinical studies are needed to confirm this.

Like gabapentin, the dosing of these other anticonvulsants typically follows the guidelines recommended for their use in the management of seizures. Patients may have markedly different analgesic responses to the various drugs (Swerdlow 1984; Swerdlow and Cundill 1981), and sequential trials may be needed to identify a useful drug.

GABA Agonists

Baclofen, a GABA agonist primarily indicated in the treatment of spasticity, has been shown to be analgesic in trigeminal neuralgia (Fromm et al. 1984). These data support the use of this drug for lancinating neuropathic pain of any type.

Systemic Local Anesthetics

Systemic administration of local anesthetic drugs is analgesic in diverse pain syndromes. In clinical practice, the use of these drugs as analgesics has been limited to neuropathic pain. In controlled clinical trials, these drugs have been effective in relieving both continuous and paroxysmal neuropathic pain (Dejgard et al. 1988; Lindstrom and Lindblom 1987). Allodynia responded better than ongoing pain in a placebo-controlled study of postherpetic neuralgia (Baranowski et al. 1999).

Neuropathic pain can be relieved, sometimes for long periods, by a brief intravenous local anesthetic infusion (Baranowski et al. 1999; Ferrante et al. 1996b; Galer et al. 1993). These data are sufficiently strong to suggest that local anesthetic infusion could be used even as a test procedure to show the neuropathic nature of a pain syndrome (Marchettini et al. 1992). Clinical trials in cancer pain have not been uniformly successful (Bruera et al. 1992; Ellemann et al. 1989), however, which suggests that some pain syndromes do not respond well or that factors related to individual pharmacokinetic and pharmacodynamic variation preclude a satisfactory outcome (Bruera et al. 1992; Galer et al. 1993). The importance of pharmacokinetic factors has been underscored by a study that identified a dose-response relationship characterized by a threshold response (Ferrante et al. 1996b).

Based on these data and a large clinical experience, a brief local anesthetic infusion may be considered as a therapeutic trial for any patient with neuropathic pain who has no contraindications to this therapy. A lidocaine infusion has been preferred in the United States. Patients with significant heart disease (such as second-

or third-degree atrioventricular block) should not be given a systemic local anesthetic, and others who could be at risk (such as the elderly and those with less serious heart disease) should undergo an appropriate cardiac evaluation before local anesthetic therapy is initiated.

A lidocaine infusion usually is administered in a dose range of 1–5 mg/kg over 20–30 minutes (Baranowski et al. 1999; Galer et al. 1993; Rowbotham et al. 1991). This dose range has not been systematically evaluated in medically ill patients, and safety considerations favor starting with a low dose in frail patients. Although one study suggested no difference in response between a low-dose and a high-dose infusion, this outcome was presumably affected by a protracted time course (2 hours) of the infusion (Baranowski et al. 1999). Given the high likelihood of dose-dependent effects (Ferrante et al. 1996b), the lack of response to a low dose should be followed by repeated infusions at progressively higher doses (Baranowski et al. 1999; Boas et al. 1982; Ferrante et al. 1996b).

An oral local anesthetic drug also may be valuable in the treatment of any type of neuropathic pain. Given the relatively limited experience with these drugs as analgesics, and their side-effect profiles, they should be considered second-line treatments for chronic neuropathic pain. An oral local anesthetic trial would be appropriate, for example, for a continuous dysesthesia that has not responded to an antidepressant or an anticonvulsant. Although limited evidence indicates that a brief intravenous local anesthetic infusion might predict the efficacy of oral administration of these drugs, experience is so limited that it is difficult to justify the withholding of an oral trial on the basis of a negative response to an intravenous infusion.

In the United States, mexiletine has been the preferred oral local anesthetic for the treatment of pain. This preference is not based on comparative trials with other local anesthetics but may be justified by a relatively better therapeutic index for serious cardiac and neurological toxicity. Alternative drugs, such as tocainide and flecainide, also have been used for neuropathic pain (Lindstrom and Lindblom 1987). Again, a history of heart disease should be addressed before therapy is initiated.

The initial dose of mexiletine should be low (e.g., 150 mg/day) and then titrated to explore the dose-response relationship for pain. Gradual dose escalation should continue until favorable effects occur, side effects become problematic, or a usual maximal daily dose of 900 mg is reached. The electrocardiogram should be monitored at higher doses. The measurement of plasma mexiletine levels may be informative to monitor compliance and toxicity. Nausea and gastric discomfort, dizziness, or tremors are frequent and can limit treatment.

NMDA Receptor Antagonists

The excitatory amino acid glutamate is released by primary afferent neurons in the dorsal horn of the spinal cord and binds to the so-called N-methyl-D-aspartate (NMDA) receptor. Activation of the NMDA receptor is part of a cascade of phenomena that are involved in the development of some neuropathic pain and opioid tolerance (Mao et al. 1995). For this reason, NMDA receptor antagonists are undergoing intensive investigation as potential analgesics.

The dissociative anesthetic ketamine is one of the commercially available NMDA receptor antagonists and has been shown to be analgesic in both controlled trials and case reports (Mathisen et al. 1995; Mercadante et al. 1995; Persson et al. 1995; Schmid et al. 1999). The clinical utility of this drug is limited by side effects, such as nightmares, hallucinations, delusions, and delirium. Although these effects are relatively unlikely to occur at the subanesthetic doses required for analgesia, which are usually in the range of 0.1–1.5 mg/kg/hour, the potential toxicity has relegated the use of ketamine to patients with severe refractory neuropathic pain.

Dextromethorphan, which is commercially available as an antitussive, also is an NMDA receptor antagonist. When coadministered with opioids, this drug attenuated tolerance to the antinociceptive effects of morphine (Mao et al. 1996; Price et al. 1994, 1996). Although 30 mg three times per day was not analgesic in two studies (McQuay et al. 1994; Mercadante et al. 1998), a controlled trial at higher doses, typically in the range of 200–400 mg/day, did produce analgesia in patients with painful diabetic neuropathy (Nelson et al. 1997). In practice, a trial of this drug may be initiated with a commercially available antitussive preparation that contains only dextromethorphan (no alcohol or guaifenesin). A reasonable maximal starting dose is 120 mg/day in three to four divided doses. This dose can be increased gradually; doses greater than 1 g have been administered safely, at least for the short term.

Other NMDA receptor antagonists are being evaluated as analgesics. Studies also are assessing the value of combination drugs that link NMDA receptor antagonists with opioids. There continues to be great promise in these analgesics, particularly for neuropathic pain.

Muscle Relaxants

Muscle relaxants are commonly used in the treatment of acute musculoskeletal pains. These drugs are often used when patients develop painful strains, spasms, or cramps. These disorders are not related to the hypertonicity that results from a lesion in the CNS, and some drugs that are useful in the treatment of true spasticity, such as baclofen and dantrolene, are not indicated for these common pains. Other drugs, specifically, diazepam and tizanidine, can be used to treat both types of conditions.

The drugs that are typically termed *muscle relaxants* are not indicated for the treatment of true spasticity. Many drugs are in this category, including orphenadrine, carisoprodol, chlorzoxazone, methocarbamol, chlorphenesin carbamate, metaxalone, and cyclobenzaprine. The mechanism of the analgesic effects produced by these drugs is unknown and probably varies. No evidence indicates that any of these drugs actually relaxes skeletal muscle. Some suppress polysynaptic reflexes in experimental preparations (Smith 1966), but this phenomenon is not associated with muscle relaxation.

Controlled studies have found analgesic efficacy greater than that of placebo for each of the muscle relaxant drugs in the treatment of musculoskeletal pain (Bercel 1977; Gold 1978). Some studies have reported analgesia above that provided by aspirin or acetaminophen or analgesia from the combination of a muscle relaxant and either aspirin or acetaminophen above that provided by the analgesic alone (Birkeland and Clawson 1968).

Based on these data, the clearest indication for these drugs is acute myofascial pain. In the absence of a published experience supporting the use of chronic administration, long-term treatment should be considered only in patients with refractory pain who show clear-cut benefits over time. The major side effects are somnolence and anticholinergic effects. Selection of a specific drug and dosing are empirical. Dose escalation beyond the usually recommended doses has not been evaluated.

Antihistamines

Controlled trials have established the analgesic potential of diphenhydramine, hydroxyzine, and orphenadrine (Birkeland and Clawson 1968; Gold 1978; Rumore and Schlichting 1986; Stambaugh and Lance 1983), and it is interesting to speculate that this effect is mediated by specific histamine receptors in endogenous pain-modulating pathways (Rumore and Schlichting 1986). As noted above, orphenadrine is used as a muscle relaxant analgesic. Other antihistamines have been combined with primary analgesics, particularly in over-the-counter preparations. Based on clinical experience, the overall analgesic efficacy of these drugs is limited.

Topical Therapies

Topical formulations of capsaicin, local anesthetics, and NSAIDs are available for pain management (Rowbotham 1994). Controlled trials support the efficacy of topical NSAIDs (Burnham et al. 1998), and several formulations are available in countries other than the United States. Additional formulations are in development and may prove useful in a wide range of painful syndromes.

The analgesic effects produced by capsaicin presumably relate to depletion of substance P from unmyelinated nociceptive primary afferent neurons. The potential efficacy of capsaicin has been suggested in both neuropathic syndromes, such as postherpetic neuralgia and painful diabetic polyneuropathy, and painful arthropathy of small joints (Tandan et al. 1992; Watson et al. 1988). Based on the safety of the commercially available formulations, a trial may be warranted in patients with neuropathic pain characterized by a prominent peripheral contribution and those with painful joints. Treatment is generally initiated with the high-concentration formulation (0.075%), which is applied three or four times daily for 1 month. Patients may experience burning at the time of application. This burning may wane with repeated use or may be attenuated with the use of an oral analgesic, a cutaneous application of lidocaine 5% ointment, or the lower-concentration formulation (0.05%).

The topical cutaneous application of local anesthetics, specifically EMLA (eutectic mixture of local anesthetics) (Ehrenstrom and Reiz 1982) and high-concentration lidocaine (Rowbotham et al. 1995), can be analgesic. EMLA is now commercially available, and a lidocaine-impregnated patch was recently approved for use in the United States. A trial of a topical local anesthetic can be considered in patients with a painful peripheral lesion or allodynia associated with neuropathic pain. Studies have not confirmed the necessity of cutaneous anesthesia to obtain analgesia.

Miscellaneous Drugs

Many other drugs have been studied as analgesics. Sympatholytic drugs have been tried in populations with complex regional pain syndrome, based on the assumption that these pains may be sympathetically maintained. Although this area is controversial (Jadad et al. 1995; Schott 1994), case reports and clinical series have suggested that phenoxybenzamine (Ghostine et al. 1984), prazosin (Abram and Lightfoot 1981), oral guanethidine (Tabira et al. 1983), and propranolol (Simson 1974) may be useful in these pains. Other drugs, specifically, a corticosteroid (Kozin et al. 1981), calcitonin (Gobelet et al. 1992), and nifedipine (Prough et al. 1985), also have been successfully administered for complex regional pain syndrome. The data best support trials of a corticosteroid and calcitonin in this condition.

Calcitonin also has been shown to be beneficial in the management of acute phantom limb pain (Jaeger and Maier 1992). With the availability of the intranasal formulation of this drug, a therapeutic trial for phantom pain, complex regional pain syndrome, and selected refractory neuropathic pain of other types is more simply administered and is often tried.

Studies in the postoperative setting have suggested analgesic potential for some benzodiazepines, including diazepam and midazolam (Miller et al. 1986; Singh et al. 1981). Clinical investigations of the effect of benzodiazepines on chronic pain have had mixed results (Fernandez et al. 1987; Yosselson-Superstine et al. 1985). A study of experimental pain in volunteers suggested that the analgesia afforded by benzodiazepines can be ascribed to their anxiolytic effects (Yang et al. 1979). With the exception of the short-term use of diazepam for acute musculoskeletal pains, and chronic administration of clonazepam for neuropathic pain, these drugs have limited utility as analgesics.

Pimozide is a neuroleptic shown to be analgesic in trigeminal neuralgia (Lechin et al. 1989). The potential for adverse effects of the neuroleptics during long-term administration suggests that the use of pimozide for lancinating neuropathic pain should be reserved for patients whose symptoms do not respond to other agents.

Drugs with sympathomimetic effects, specifically, dextroamphetamine, methylphenidate, and caffeine, also are analgesic (Bruera et al. 1987; Forrest et al. 1977; Laska et al. 1984). Caffeine is commonly added to combination products used to treat headache, and both dextroamphetamine and methylphenidate are used to reverse opioid-induced sedation and provide coanalgesic effects in patients with cancer pain.

Opioid Analgesics

The opioids are the most useful analgesics available, yet their appropriate medical use is problematic because of a pervasive lack of knowledge about their true risks and benefits and the unfortunate stigmatization that follows from their association with addiction and abuse. Opioids are underused in conditions for which they are recommended as first-line therapy, such as cancer pain, and their long-term use in chronic nonmalignant pain is controversial (Ward et al. 1993).

Basic and Clinical Opioid Pharmacology

The analgesic activity of opioids is primarily a result of binding to opioid receptors in the CNS. These compounds mimic the actions of endogenous opioids (endorphins) at multiple types of opioid receptors, including μ, δ, and κ. Opioids have both presynaptic and postsynaptic inhibitory effects, which are mediated by a second-messenger system that uses a guanine nucleotide-binding protein (G protein) (Dickenson 1994). A very important part of the presynaptic opioid inhibitory activity on pain pathways takes place at the spinal cord level, where opioids inhibit nociceptive afferents. Peripheral opioid receptors also have been identified on sensory nerves and cells of the immune system (Stein 1994), and a peripheral mechanism may contribute to opioid analgesia (Dalsgaard et al. 1994; Joshi et al. 1993; Stein et al. 1993).

Depending on their receptor interactions, the opioids can be classified as antagonists, agonist-antagonists, or agonists (Hoskin and Hanks 1991). The *antagonists,* including naloxone, naltrexone, and nalmefene, bind to opioid receptors but produce no opioid activity. The *agonist-antagonists* include a mixed agonist-antagonist subclass that produces agonist effects at a non-μ receptor and antagonist effects at the μ receptor and a partial agonist subclass that is an agonist at the μ receptor but produces a lesser maximal effect than a full agonist. The mixed drugs include butorphanol, nalbuphine, pentazocine, and dezocine; buprenorphine is a partial agonist. All the agonist-antagonists have limited utility in chronic pain because of a ceiling effect for analgesia, a relatively high side-effect liability for some of these drugs, the possibility of inducing withdrawal in patients with previous significant opioid exposure, and the limited availability of oral formulations.

Pure μ *agonists* are the preferred agents for the treatment of acute and chronic nociceptive pain (Table 2–3). These drugs have no ceiling effect for analgesia. Pain relief and other effects increase proportionately with the dose. Nonanalgesic CNS effects, mainly sedation and respiratory depression, are the most relevant treatment-limiting toxicities.

Opioid Responsiveness

Opioid responsiveness is a term that has been proposed to describe the probability that adequate analgesia (satisfactory relief without intolerable and unmanageable side effects) can be attained during

Table 2–3. Conversion table for opioid analgesics used for the treatment of chronic pain

| Drug | Dose (mg) equianalgesic to morphine 10 mg im[a] | | Half-life duration | | Comment |
	po	im	(hours)	(hours)	
Morphine	20–30[b,c]	10	2–3	2–4	
Oxycodone[c]	20	—	2–3	3–4	
Hydromorphone	7.5	1.5	2–3	2–4	Potency may be greater (iv hydromorphone to iv morphine = 3:1 rather than 6.7:1) during prolonged use.
Methadone	20	10	12–190	4–12	Although a 1:1 iv ratio with morphine was found in a single-dose study, with chronic dosing, a large dose reduction (75%–90%) is needed when switching to methadone.
Oxymorphone	10	1 (rectal)	2–3	2–4	Available in rectal and injectable formulations.
Levorphanol	4	2	12–15	4–6	

Table 2–3. Conversion table for opioid analgesics used for the treatment of chronic pain (*continued*)

Drug	Dose (mg) equianalgesic to morphine 10 mg im[a]		Half-life duration		Comment
	po	im	(hours)	(hours)	
Fentanyl	—	—	7–12	—	Can be administered as a continuous iv or sq infusion; based on clinical experience, 100 µg/hour is roughly equianalgesic to iv morphine 4 mg/hour.
Fentanyl TTS	—	—	16–24	48–72	Based on clinical experience, 100 mg/hour is roughly equianalgesic to iv morphine 4 µg/hour. A ratio of oral morphine–to–transdermal fentanyl of 70:1 also may be used clinically.

Note. im = intramuscular; po = oral; iv = intravenous; sq = subcutaneous.

[a]Studies to determine equianalgesic doses of opioids have used morphine by the im route. The im and iv routes are considered to be equivalent, and iv is the most common route used in clinical practice.

[b]Although the po-to-im morphine ratio was 6:1 in a single-dose study, other observations indicate a ratio of 2–3:1 with repeated administration.

[c]po morphine and oxycodone slow-release preparation are available, which provide extended plasma levels allowing dosing every 8–12 hours (morphine and oxycodone CR) and dosing every 24 hours (morphine SR).

Source. Adapted from Derby S, Chin J, Portenoy RK: "Systemic Opioid Therapy for Chronic Cancer Pain: Practical Guidelines for Converting Drugs and Routes of Administration." *CNS Drugs* 9(2):99–109, 1998. Used with permission.

dose titration. Factors that appear to reduce opioid responsiveness include a neuropathic mechanism for the pain, the presence of breakthrough pain, a high level of psychological distress, and the need for rapid dose escalation after therapy is initiated (Bruera et al. 1989b; Cherny et al. 1994; Mercadante et al. 1992). Responsiveness cannot be accurately predicted in any specific case, however, and in most situations, the responsiveness to a particular opioid can be determined only through gradual dose escalation until relief is adequate or intolerable and unmanageable side effects supervene (Jadad et al. 1992; McQuay et al. 1992; Portenoy et al. 1990). The most important corollary of this observation is that an opioid regimen cannot be considered ineffective unless the dose has been slowly increased to treatment-limiting toxicity.

Organ Toxicity and Immune Effects

Chronic opioid therapy does not produce major organ damage (Kreek 1978; Kreek et al. 1972). A dysimmune effect is possible, but the clinical relevance of this is unclear. In animal models, acute opioid exposure can alter both humoral and cell-mediated immune function (Molitor et al. 1992; Shavit et al. 1984; Weber et al. 1987). Prolonged morphine administration (up to 42 days) in a swine model significantly diminished cell-mediated immunity (Molitor et al. 1992) but did not affect humoral immune responses. In other studies, however, lower morphine doses (Shavit et al. 1987) and sustained treatment with methadone (Ochshorn et al. 1990) had no effect on natural killer cell activity. Although opioids may reduce the $CD4^+$ T-cell number in humans (Donohoe and Falek 1988), there have been no clinical observations that relate to this finding. In summary, no evidence indicates that the immune effects of opioid drugs have adverse clinical consequences, and the potential for these effects has not altered guidelines for opioid administration in practice.

Side Effects

The most important opioid side effects are constipation, nausea or vomiting, and sedation or mental clouding. Tolerance develops to many side effects, usually during the initial weeks of therapy. Studies in methadone maintenance patients reported that approximately 10%–20% complain of persistent constipation, insomnia, and decreased sexual function, and a somewhat higher percentage report persistent sweating (Kreek 1978). In the cancer population, constipation is the most problematic long-term side effect.

Strategies for the treatment of common opioid side effects are summarized in Table 2–4. Cognitive impairment is probably the most worrisome of these effects because of the potential to further impair function. Although additional studies of this phenomenon are needed, clinical experience and some empirical data suggest that adverse cognitive effects are generally pronounced after acute dosing or dose increases but decline with chronic administration (Bruera et al. 1989a; Vainio et al. 1995). When cognitive changes persist, they are usually mild (Banning and Sjogren 1990; Haertzen and Hooks 1969; Hendler et al. 1980; Lombardo et al. 1976; Mc-Nairy et al. 1984; Sjogren and Banning 1989). This outcome must be balanced against the potential cognitive impairment that can occur from uncontrolled pain, particularly in the medically ill.

Tolerance

Tolerance refers to the phenomenon in which repetitive exposure to a drug results in a decreasing effect of a given dose or the need for a higher dose to maintain the same effect (Foley 1993; Jaffe 1985; Portenoy 1994b). Although animal models show that tolerance to the antinociceptive effects of opioids occurs rapidly, the situation in humans is far more complex (Cochin and Kornetsky 1964). Tolerance to the nonanalgesic effects, including somnolence, mental clouding, nausea, and respiratory depressant effects, usually occurs within days to weeks. This phenomenon allows safe escalation of the opioid dose. Clinically, tolerance to these side effects is beneficial and increases the likelihood that a favorable balance between analgesia and side effects will be attained during dose escalation.

In the clinical setting, the development of tolerance to the analgesic effect of opioids is confounded by the ongoing pain. In contrast to the findings in experimental paradigms (Houde 1985; Houde et al. 1966), patients without progressive disease who are administered an opioid typically achieve stable dosing that extends for a prolonged period (Brescia et al. 1992; Foley 1993;

Table 2–4. Common strategies to manage opioid side effects

Constipation
Best managed with a combination of cathartic and stool softener
Osmotic agents can be useful (lactulose)
Refractory constipation can be treated with a trial of oral naloxone

Nausea, Vomiting
Metoclopramide 10 mg three times a day
Prochlorperazine 10 mg three times a day
Haloperidol 1–2 mg/day
Scopolamine patch
Change route of administration
Switch opioid

Sedation
Methylphenidate 5 mg twice a day
Pemoline 18.75–37.50 mg twice a day

Delirium
Haloperidol (neurological/psychiatric opinion needed)
Switch opioid

Myoclonus
Clonazepam 0.5 mg three times a day
Switch opioid

Urinary retention
Cholinomimetic drugs

Respiratory depression
Naloxone 0.4 mg diluted in 10 cc saline intravenous push of 1 mL
  until respiratory rate recovers is useful to monitor oxygen saturation.
  Witdrawal may be precipitated if the dose is not carefully titrated.

Source. Reprinted from Caraceni A, Portenoy RK: "Pain," in *Clinical Neurology.* Edited by Griggs RC, Joynt RJ. Philadelphia, PA, Lippincott-Raven (in press). Used with permission.

Houde 1985; Houde et al. 1966; Kanner and Foley 1981; Schug et al. 1992). When dose escalation is necessary, an alternative explanation (typically, worsening of the underlying disease) usually can be found (Gonzales et al. 1991). For this reason, the need for dose escalation should usually prompt reevaluation of the underlying syndrome.

Physical Dependence

Physical dependence is characterized by the development of an abstinence syndrome following sudden discontinuation of therapy, reduction in dose, or administration of an antagonist drug (Jaffe 1985). This phenomenon is distinct from addiction (see below), and it is never appropriate to use the term *addicted* to describe the capacity for abstinence.

The risk of withdrawal is presumed to exist whenever repeated doses of an opioid have been administered for more than a few days. Abstinence should be prevented by avoiding abrupt dose reduction and opioid antagonist drug administration. When therapy must be terminated, gradual dose tapering is preferred (Buckley et al. 1986; Kanner and Foley 1981).

Although physical dependence should pose no difficulties during long-term opioid therapy as long as abstinence is avoided, there have been theoretical concerns that subtle abstinence phenomena may perpetuate pain or disability in some patients with chronic noncancer pain (Brodner and Taub 1978; Portenoy 1994a; Portenoy and Payne 1997; Schofferman 1993; Ziegler 1994). This concept has not been confirmed.

Addiction

Common definitions of *addiction* incorporate reference to tolerance and dependence and can be confusing when considering patients who are receiving opioids as prescribed therapy for an appropriate medical indication (Jaffe 1985; Passik and Portenoy 1998; Portenoy and Payne 1997). A task force of the American Medical Association defined addiction as a chronic disorder characterized by compulsive use and physical, psychological, or social harm to the user (Rinaldi et al. 1988). This definition emphasizes that addiction is a psychological and behavioral syndrome with several fundamental features: 1) loss of control over drug use, 2) compulsive drug use, and 3) continued use despite harm. In treating pain patients, addiction is suggested by the development of aberrant drug-related behaviors consistent with these features (Passik and Portenoy 1998; Portenoy and Payne 1997).

Concern about the potential for iatrogenic addiction has been reinforced by surveys of patients with chronic nonmalignant pain referred to pain clinics, which identified high rates of aberrant drug-related behavior (Chabal et al. 1992; Finlayson et al. 1986a, 1986b). The addiction rates reported in these programs, which ranged from 3.2% to 18.9% (Fishbain et al. 1992), are much higher than those reported in other types of surveys, which suggest very low addiction rates in general hospital populations (Porter and Jick 1980), patients with burn pain (Perry and Heidrich 1982), and patients with headache (Medina and Diamond 1977). In the cancer pain population, extensive experience suggests that addiction can be discounted unless the patient has a history of drug abuse.

Although the risk of iatrogenic addiction in patients without a history of drug abuse is likely to be very low, all patients must be carefully assessed on an ongoing basis for the occurrence of aberrant drug-related behavior. If this type of behavior occurs, a further evaluation is needed to establish a diagnosis and a care plan that includes management of both the drug use and the pain. The treatment of pain in patients with a known history of chemical dependency is particularly challenging (Passik and Portenoy 1998).

Opioids in the Management of Cancer Pain

Opioid administration is the mainstay of pain management in cancer. Although as many as 90% of patients benefit from optimally administered opioid therapy (Mercadante 1999; Schug et al. 1990; Takeda 1986; Ventafridda et al. 1987b), undertreatment continues in most practice settings (Cleeland et al. 1994). Improved use of current techniques for opioid therapy is one of the goals of the treatment guidelines for cancer pain published by the U.S. Agency for Health Care Policy and Research (Jacox et al. 1994).

The WHO Ladder Approach

The feasibility and benefits of the World Health Organization (WHO; 1996) guidelines for the management of cancer pain, which are known as the *analgesic ladder approach* (Figure 2–1), have been evaluated in large open trials (Mercadante 1999; Schug et al. 1990; Takeda 1986; Ventafridda et al. 1987b). According to this approach, patients with mild to moderate cancer-related pain first should receive an NSAID or acetaminophen. If needed, this drug is combined with an adjuvant drug to provide additional analgesia or to treat a different symptom (either a side effect of the analgesic or a coexisting symptom other than pain). Relatively few patients with chronic cancer-related pain remain on this first "rung" of the analgesic ladder.

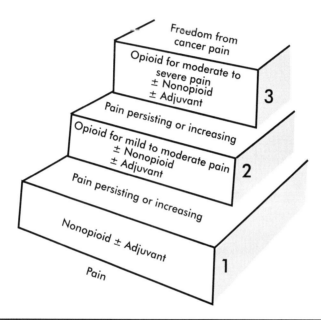

Figure 2–1. Analgesic ladder approach for drug selection for the management of cancer pain, as developed by a committee of the World Health Organization.

Source. Reprinted from World Health Organization: *Cancer Pain Relief,* 2nd Edition, With a Guide to Opioid Availability. Geneva, World Health Organization, 1996. Used with permission.

Patients with moderate or severe pain should receive primarily an opioid-based regimen. Specifically, those with moderate pain or continued pain despite treatment with a nonopioid analgesic should be given an opioid conventionally used for moderate pain (previously termed a *weak* opioid). This drug is often combined with an NSAID and may be administered with an adjuvant drug, if indicated. Those with severe pain or continued pain despite administration of an opioid for moderate pain should be given an opioid conventionally used for severe pain (previously termed a *strong* opioid). This drug also may be combined with an NSAID or an adjuvant drug, as indicated.

In the United States, the opioids used for moderate pain include codeine, hydrocodone, dihydrocodeine, oxycodone (combined with aspirin or acetaminophen), propoxyphene, and occasionally meperidine. Although these pure μ agonists do not have a true ceiling dose, the doses used are sufficient for managing moderate pain in the relatively opioid-naive patient. Hydrocodone and dihydrocodeine also are available only in tablets that contain acetaminophen or aspirin and cannot be given in quantities that exceed the maximal safe amount of acetaminophen (e.g., 4–6 g/day of acetaminophen).

The opioids used to treat moderate pain that are available in single entity formulations could potentially be used at higher doses to treat more severe pain. Oxycodone, which is now available in a controlled-release formulation, is commonly used for this purpose. Although propoxyphene and meperidine are available in single entity formulations, dose escalation is not recommended because of the risk of enhanced toxicity from the accumulation of toxic metabolites (Kaiko et al. 1983). The possibility of normeperidine toxicity suggests that meperidine generally should not be used for chronic pain.

In most cases, the treatment of moderate pain in a patient with limited or no prior exposure to opioids involves the administration of a combination product containing an opioid conventionally used on the second rung of the analgesic ladder (usually codeine, oxycodone, hydrocodone, dihydrocodeine, or propoxyphene) and either aspirin or acetaminophen. The dose can be increased, if needed, until maximal doses of the coanalgesic are reached (e.g., two to three tablets every 4 hours of a combination product containing 325 mg of acetaminophen per tablet).

Traditionally, morphine was selected first when an opioid for severe pain was needed. This choice was based on extensive worldwide experience and the availability of numerous formulations, including a sustained-release form with a duration of 12–24 hours. The availability of other long-acting drugs in developed countries offers many other options. Morphine has no inherent advantage, and a different drug may be selected. Chronic pain is now often treated with oxycodone, hydromorphone, fentanyl, methadone, and levorphanol. Given the very large intraindividual variability in opioid responsiveness, sequential trials are commonly needed to identify the most salutary drug. A switch from one drug or route to another should be guided by a table of equianalgesic doses (Table 2–3); the dose of the new drug or route is typically reduced by 30%–50% (and as much as 90% when the switch is to methadone) to avoid unanticipated toxicity. Once a drug is selected, well-accepted dosing guidelines (Table 2–5) (Jacox et al. 1994), which emphasize individualization of the dose, are likely to yield a favorable response.

Route of Administration

In most cases, the oral route of administration is preferred for the management of chronic cancer pain because of its safety, economy, and acceptability to patients. The transdermal route, which is available for the highly lipophilic opioid fentanyl, has become widely used, however, and is particularly helpful for many patients who cannot swallow or absorb an orally administered opioid, patients who are noncompliant with oral drugs or would prefer an alternative, and patients who have failed other opioid trials and may benefit from a trial of fentanyl.

Intravenous or subcutaneous infusions are facilitated by the use of portable ambulatory infusion devices (Swanson et al. 1989). Patients who are unable to swallow or absorb opioids also can be managed in the ambulatory setting for long periods with this approach. Devices that include a patient-controlled analgesia system may be very useful for patients who have frequent and severe breakthrough pain.

Opioids can be administered via catheters into the epidural or subarachnoid spinal spaces (see subsection "Intraspinal Drug Administration" below). Spinal administration usually is considered for patients who have intolerable side effects from systemic opioids. Spinal drug administration may provide the same level of analgesia at lower opioid doses (Plummer et al. 1991; Waldman 1990).

Table 2–5.   Oral morphine or equivalent pure agonist opioid initial dosing guidelines

Initial dose
15–30 mg of immediate-release morphine every 4 hours or equivalent
30–90 mg of slow-release morphine every 12 hours
Lower doses are used in elderly or frail patients.

Titrate dose to effect
Increase total daily dose by at least 30%–50% of previous dose every
  24 hours until pain relief is satisfactory or excessive unmanageable
  side effects occur.
Maximum recommended dose is immaterial; individual variability can
  be >10-fold.
Dose may need to be reduced after effective alternative pain-relieving
  procedure (e.g., radiotherapy).

Fixed around-the-clock dosing
Advantageous in most patients; allows pain relief and nighttime sleep
  and prevents pain recurrence.

As-needed dosing
Pain relief is often uneven, and breakthrough pain is very common;
  in most cases, as-needed doses with a short-acting opioid are offered
  every 2 hours. Doses should be equal to 5%–15% of daily require-
  ments.

Side effects management
Explain potential main side effects to the patient; side effects are
  treatable.
Give prophylactic therapy for constipation in predisposed patients.

Source.   Reprinted with permission from Caraceni A, Portenoy RK: "Pain," in
Clinical Neurology. Edited by Griggs RC, Joynt RJ. Philadelphia, PA, Lippincott-
Raven (in press). Used with permission.

Opioids in the Management of Chronic Nonmalignant Pain

Experience in the use of chronic opioid therapy for refractory nonmalignant pain syndromes is growing. Several case series and
successful clinical reports have reinforced this trend (Brena and
Sanders 1991; Chabal et al. 1992; Gourlay and Cherry 1991; Merry
et al. 1992; Portenoy and Foley 1986; Portenoy and Payne 1997).
For example, a prospective survey of 100 patients with diverse
neuropathic or nociceptive pain syndromes found that dihydro-

codeine, buprenorphine, or morphine provided greater than 50% analgesia to 51 patients and 25%–50% analgesia to 28 patients at a 1-month assessment (Zenz et al. 1992). In this group of patients, treatment was associated with an improvement on the Karnofsky Performance Status Scale, with the largest improvement noted among those with the greatest relief of pain, and no incidents of serious toxicity or aberrant drug-related behaviors occurred. Recent controlled clinical trials confirmed that opioids have analgesic effects in chronic nonmalignant pain, even when pain is caused by a neuropathic mechanism (Moulin et al. 1996; Watson and Babul 1998).

Guidelines for opioid therapy in chronic nonmalignant pain are empirical and evolving (Table 2–6) (France et al. 1984; Portenoy 1994a; Portenoy and Payne 1997). These guidelines reflect the view that opioids are not a panacea for chronic pain and, indeed, can contribute to poor outcomes in some cases. Increasing comfort with this therapy on the part of clinicians supports the role of a therapeutic opioid trial, which can be discontinued if negative outcomes exceed benefits. These treatment trials should incorporate dose adjustment and careful monitoring of clinically relevant end points, including pain relief, side effects, functional status, the willingness to engage in other components of therapy, and the development of aberrant drug-related behaviors. If long-term therapy is attempted, these end points should be monitored over time. Patients should be informed about the controversial nature of this approach, and written or oral consent should be obtained. Consultation with a specialist in pain management may be useful in deciding whether to continue a trial.

Anesthesiological Therapies

Anesthesiological techniques include neuraxial drug administration, neural blockade, and invasive neurostimulatory approaches. These therapies usually are considered after more conservative approaches have failed.

Intraspinal Drug Administration

Long-term intraspinal opioid administration is a well-accepted strategy for the management of cancer pain and chronic nonma-

Table 2–6.   Proposed guidelines in the management of opioid therapy for chronic nonmalignant pain

1. The role of opioid therapy is evolving. In some cases, it should be considered only after all other reasonable attempts at analgesia have failed. In others, an early trial is appropriate.

2. The use of opioid therapy in an individual with a history of substance abuse is clinically complex and should be approached with great care. The inclusion of a clinician experienced in addictions evaluation and treatment is recommended in such instances.

3. A single practitioner should take primary responsibility for treatment.

4. Patients should give informed consent before starting therapy; points to be covered include recognition of the low risk of true addiction as an outcome, potential for cognitive impairment with the drug alone and in combination with sedative-hypnotics, likelihood that physical dependence will occur (abstinence syndrome possible with acute discontinuation), and understanding by female patients that children born while the mother is taking opioid therapy will likely be physically dependent at birth.

5. After drug selection, doses should be given around the clock; several weeks should be agreed on as the period of initial dose titration, and although improvement in function should be continually stressed, all should agree to at least partial analgesia as the appropriate goal of therapy.

6. Failure to achieve at least partial analgesia at relatively low initial doses in the nontolerant patient raises questions about the potential treatability of the pain syndrome with opioids.

7. Capitalizing on improved analgesia by gains in physical and social function should be emphasized; opioid therapy should be considered complementary to other analgesic and rehabilitative approaches.

8. In addition to the daily dose determined initially, patients should be permitted to escalate the dose transiently on days of increased pain; two methods are acceptable: 1) prescription of an additional 4–6 "rescue doses" to be taken as needed during the month and 2) instruction that 1 or 2 extra doses may be taken on any day but must be followed by an equal reduction in dose on subsequent days.

Table 2–6. Proposed guidelines in the management of opioid therapy for chronic nonmalignant pain *(continued)*

9. Initially, patients must be seen and drugs prescribed at least monthly. When patients are stable, less-frequent visits may be acceptable.

10. Exacerbations of pain not effectively treated by transient, small increases in dose are best managed in the hospital, where dose escalation, if appropriate, can be observed closely, and return to baseline doses can be accomplished in a controlled environment.

11. Evidence of drug hoarding, acquisition of drugs from other physicians, uncontrolled dose escalation, or other aberrant behaviors must be carefully assessed. In some cases, tapering and discontinuation of opioid therapy will be necessary. Other patients may appropriately continue therapy within rigid guidelines. Consideration should be given to consultation with an addiction medicine specialist.

12. At each visit, assessment should specifically address

    a) Comfort (degree of analgesia)
    b) Opioid-related side effects
    c) Functional status (physical and psychosocial)
    d) Existence of aberrant drug-related behaviors

13. Use of self-report instruments may be helpful but should not be required.

14. Documentation is essential, and the medical record should specifically address comfort, function, side effects, and the occurrence of aberrant behaviors repeatedly during the course of therapy.

Source. Adapted with permission from Portenoy RK: "Opioid Therapy for Chronic Nonmalignant Pain: Current Status," in *Progress in Pain Research and Management, Vol 1: Pharmacological Approaches to the Treatment of Chronic Pain: New Concepts and Critical Issues.* Edited by Fields HL, Liebeskind JC. Seattle, WA, IASP Press, 1994a, pp. 247–288. Used with permission.

lignant pain (Arner et al. 1988; Cousins et al. 1988a; Gestin et al. 1997; Plummer et al. 1991; Waldman 1990). This approach allows the use of relatively low opioid doses to achieve therapeutic effects. This may improve the balance between analgesia and side effects and potentially yield greater efficacy in syndromes that respond poorly to systemic therapy as a result of the onset of dose-related side effects. A trial of intraspinal opioid therapy should be considered only in selected patients who experience an unfavorable balance between analgesia and side effects during systemic opioid therapy.

Either epidural or subarachnoid infusion can be used in long-term therapy (Waldman and Coombs 1989). A successful trial with a temporary catheter is prerequisite for implantation of a more permanent system. Technical complications of implanted intraspinal devices include migration, kinking, breaking, and disconnecting. Epidural catheters can be blocked by local fibrosis. Infectious complications are possible and vary with the different delivery systems (Waldman et al. 1993). Minor skin or track infections may be managed without removing the catheter. Epidural abscesses during long-term epidural therapy and meningitis during subarachnoid treatment are rare if very careful preventive measures are used.

Although comparative studies of epidural and subarachnoid administration are very limited, it is now generally accepted that patients with life expectancies greater than 3–6 months are better managed with a totally implanted subarachnoid system. Whatever the approach, treatment requires ongoing monitoring by a knowledgeable clinician (Ferrante et al. 1996a).

In some difficult pain syndromes, the combination of an opioid plus a local anesthetic or clonidine may improve outcomes (Du Pen et al. 1992; Eisenach et al. 1995; Hogan et al. 1991; Sjoberg et al. 1991). Although experience with this therapy is greatest in the cancer population, the use of combined therapy for nonmalignant pain is becoming more common.

Temporary Neural Blockade

Neural blockade with a local anesthetic may be used to provide temporary relief, to determine the afferent neural pathways that are involved in sustaining the pain, and, in the case of cancer pain, to clarify the potential benefit of a subsequent neurolytic block. In some circumstances, a local anesthetic block can produce prolonged pain relief. This outcome is most notable in those patients in whom so-called sympathetically maintained pain is identified by virtue of a highly favorable response to sympathetic nerve blocks. Sympathetically maintained pain, a subtype of neuropathic pain, can be a feature of any pain syndrome but appears to be disproportionately represented in the population of patients who develop regional pain associated with autonomic or trophic changes or complex regional pain syndrome. When complex regional pain syndrome is diagnosed, early sympathetic nerve block should be considered, notwithstanding continued controversy about the definition of sympathetically maintained pain and the role of this intervention (Max and Gilron 1999).

Early use of a temporary local anesthetic block also may be indicated if strong evidence indicates a peripheral "generator" for the pain. For example, if the pain is believed to be related to the development of a neuroma, local anesthetic injection may be both diagnostic and therapeutic.

Trigger Point Injection

Pains that originate from focal areas in muscle or connective tissue are common. When focal point tenderness is found in the muscle or connective tissue, injection of a local anesthetic into the affected region can sometimes yield analgesia that outlasts the duration of the drug itself. Injections usually are most strongly considered if discrete trigger points can be identified through palpation of the painful muscle.

Chemical Neurolysis

Permanent nerve lesioning with alcohol or phenol injections (neurolysis) usually is considered only in patients with limited life expectancies who benefit temporarily from local anesthetic injections and have failed nondestructive approaches. If neurolysis is being considered, the pain must be well localized, and the block must not compromise strength or sphincter function.

The most common type of neurolytic somatic nerve block is chemical rhizotomy, which can be performed through instillation of the neurolytic solution into either the epidural or the subarachnoid space (Cousins et al. 1988b). One of the most useful rhizotomies is the "saddle" block for perineal cancer pain, which may be considered for those patients with preexisting sphincter dysfunction (Ventafridda et al. 1979). The aim in rhizotomy is to denervate specific dermatomes. Case series suggest that these blocks can produce favorable outcomes in approximately two-thirds of patients, with a duration of relief that typically exceeds 1 month and often extends to more than 3 months. If the procedure is expertly performed, then complications should occur in fewer than 15% of patients (Jain and Patt 1993; Ventafridda et al. 1976). Some patients dislike the sensory dysfunction that is the expected outcome of the procedure, and, rarely, a dysesthetic pain can develop as a consequence of the nerve injury.

Neurolytic celiac plexus is widely used and can provide good analgesia to as many as three-quarters of patients with pain due to pancreatic cancer (Caraceni and Portenoy 1996). This technique also can relieve pain caused by other tumors involving the upper abdominal region and the retroperitoneum, provided the pain is dependent on afferents that travel through the plexus. The common adverse effects (temporary orthostatic hypotension and cramping or diarrhea caused by increased GI motility) are usually mild and self-limiting. More severe complications, such as neuritis, hemorrhage, renal injury, and paraplegia, are very uncommon when the procedure is performed appropriately, but the potential for these complications should be appreciated (Caraceni and Portenoy 1996). Neurolytic celiac plexus block should not be used for the pain of chronic pancreatitis or other nonmalignant abdominal lesions because of the potential for complications and because the overall efficacy appears far lower than that observed in populations with cancer.

Hypogastric plexus block has been performed for pain originating from pelvic neoplasms (de Leon Casasola et al. 1993), and neurolysis of the ganglion impar (Walther's ganglion), which is situated at the sacrococcygeal junction, has been used to treat pain originating from injury to visceral structures at the pelvic floor. Clinical experience with these techniques is very limited.

Surgical Therapies

Surgery is often attempted to correct structural problems that are believed to be the source of the pain. In some situations, this intervention is highly successful. Joint replacement for painful arthropathy and resection of a painful neuroma (Burchiel 1997), for example, can have dramatically favorable effects in appropriately selected patients.

Surgical approaches intended to alter pain pathways directly also have been used as primary analgesic interventions. The use of these approaches has declined steadily as noninvasive and invasive but nondestructive therapies have advanced (Ventafridda 1989). The importance of ethical considerations when the goal of the treatment is a permanent neurological lesion also has been highlighted as a reason for caution (Lipton 1987).

Surgical interruption or resection of peripheral nerves (peripheral neurectomy, surgical rhizotomy) has been largely supplanted by nondestructive interventions, such as intraspinal drug infusion. Resection of neuroma and surgical sympathectomy are still commonly performed if a local anesthetic injection strongly suggests that permanent lesioning might produce prolonged benefits. Trigeminal neurectomy or rhizotomy is occasionally considered for those patients with trigeminal neuralgia refractory to pharmacological treatments, again only if profound analgesia can be shown following a diagnostic local anesthetic block.

Many surgical procedures have been designed by functional neurosurgeons to try to intercept the central nervous pathways involved in pain (Table 2–7) (Portenoy 1998). The most useful procedure is cordotomy. In this technique, the spinothalamic tract is coagulated with a radiofrequency lesion or sectioned via an open procedure. Percutaneous radiofrequency cordotomy, an ambulatory procedure that does not require general anesthesia, is now preferred (Ischia et al. 1985). More than two-thirds of appropriately selected patients with pain from unilateral nociceptive lesions can be expected to attain relief immediately after cordotomy (Ischia et al. 1985; Tasker and North 1997). Patients with neuropathic pain, specifically those with deafferentation syndromes, appear to benefit less often than those with nociceptive pain (Tasker and North 1997). Pain relief usually lasts for at least months, and sometimes as long as many years, unless the etiology of the pain progresses to involve a site outside of the denervated region.

Complications from cordotomy are occasionally severe. Death can result from respiratory failure if the lesion impairs the ipsilat-

Table 2–7. Central nervous system procedures that have been designed for chronic pain management

Approach	Comment
Percutaneous cordotomy	Usually performed in the awake patient via a lateral approach at C1-2; most common procedure currently performed
Open cordotomy	Sometimes used if percutaneous procedure is not feasible or bilateral thoracic cordotomy would be preferable lesion
Dorsal root entry zone lesion	Performed for brachial plexus avulsion pain (limited experience with postherpetic neuralgia)
Midline commissural myelotomy	Open procedure that can produce bilateral, segmental analgesia; dysesthesias appear to be a relatively common complication
Stereotactic central myelotomy	Stereotactic lesion with limited longitudinal extent placed at an upper cervical cord level; experience is limited but appears capable of providing analgesia to any caudal site; rarely considered
Cingulotomy	Performed stereotactically; can produce analgesia in the setting of diffuse or multifocal pain; rarely considered
Hypothalamotomy	Experience limited, but effects appear similar to those of cingulotomy; rarely considered
Thalamotomy	Various nuclei have been targeted with stereotactic approaches; medial nuclei and pulvinar are the preferred sites; rarely considered
Other brain stem tractotomies	Mesencephalotomy, pontine spinothalamic tractotomy, and trigeminal tractotomy have been performed as open or stereotactic procedures; denervation can be produced anywhere in the head or body; experience is limited; rarely considered
Hypophysectomy	Pituitary can be ablated through an open procedure or transphenoidally by using alcohol instillation, radiofrequency lesioning, or other approaches; large experience suggests benefit for diffuse or multifocal pain; mechanism not known

Source.   Reprinted from Portenoy RK: *Contemporary Diagnosis and Management of Pain in Oncologic and AIDS Patients,* 2nd Edition. Newtown, PA, Handbooks in Healthcare, 1998, pp. 176–177. Used with permission, Handbooks in Health Care Co.

eral diaphragm and the contralateral lung is significantly diseased. Postcordotomy dysesthesia, a central pain syndrome, is a late complication of cordotomy and can be very difficult to treat (Tasker and North 1997). Some patients develop "mirror pain" ipsilateral to the cordotomy. This pain is typically focal (sometimes representing a worsening of a prior mild pain), may be transitory or persistent, and may or may not have an associated identifiable pathology. As many as 10% of the patients who undergo cordotomy experience weakness of the leg ipsilateral to the lesion, and as many as 25% report bladder dysfunction; sexual dysfunction is also possible in men. Bilateral cordotomy is associated with a higher risk of weakness and bladder dysfunction, and the likelihood of long-lasting complications is higher than with unilateral cordotomy (Sanders and Zurmond 1995).

These potential complications suggest that the use of cordotomy should be limited to patients with advanced diseases who have not responded to more conservative measures. Like other neurolytic approaches, the use of cordotomy has declined markedly as the knowledge of analgesic pharmacology has improved and other nondestructive techniques have become available.

Dorsal root entry zone lesion is another surgical approach directed at the spinal cord. This lesion appears to be highly effective for patients with pain caused by an avulsed nerve plexus, particularly the brachial plexus (Nashold and Ostdahl 1979). The lesion is placed in the substantia gelatinosa at the dermatomal level corresponding to the painful area.

Other interventions on the spinal cord, brain stem, brain, and hypophysis have been developed (Berkley 1997; Gybels 1997). These procedures are rarely attempted now.

Neurostimulatory Therapies

Stimulation of the nervous system may produce analgesia. The best known application of this principle is transcutaneous electrical nerve stimulation (TENS). Other approaches include counterirritation (systematic rubbing of the painful part), acupuncture, percutaneous electrical nerve stimulation, dorsal column stimulation, and deep brain stimulation.

TENS and acupuncture are widely used, and both surveys and partially controlled trials of these approaches have been done. Meta-analyses of these data have not established efficacy (Agency for Health Care Policy and Research 1992; Ter Riet et al. 1990), and the likelihood of a strong placebo effect with interventions of this type must be acknowledged. Nevertheless, a substantial proportion of patients report some analgesia and, given the safety of these techniques and the small chance of prolonged benefit, a trial usually is justified. An adequate trial of TENS typically involves several weeks, during which the patient should experiment with different electrode placements and stimulation parameters (Gersh and Wolf 1985).

Dorsal column stimulation appears to benefit a subset of carefully selected patients with chronic nonmalignant pain (North et al. 1993). The most common indication has been chronic low back pain following spinal surgery; other indications have included refractory neuropathic pains, including those related to spinal cord injury and peripheral nerve injury. Although the experience in medically ill populations is minimal, dorsal column stimulation might be considered on theoretical grounds as an option for refractory neuropathic pain in patients with relatively long life expectancies and good performance status.

Deep brain stimulation at any of numerous sites has been used for decades to manage small numbers of patients with refractory pain. A recent review suggested that almost 60% of patients benefit substantially, and serious complications occur in fewer than 5% (Young and Rinaldi 1997). The need for an experienced clinician to implement this treatment, combined with a growing number of interventions for refractory pain that are perceived to be less invasive, has relegated brain stimulation to a rarely considered option.

Psychological Approaches

The comprehensive assessment of the patient with chronic pain must clarify psychological factors that potentially contribute to the pain, influence coping and adaptation, or are relevant comorbidities. Based on this assessment, the clinician can judge the utility of psychotherapy or psychotropic drugs.

Specific cognitive and behavioral approaches have become widely accepted in the management of pain (Gatchel and Turk 1996; Turk et al. 1983). Cognitive approaches include relaxation training, distraction techniques, hypnosis, and biofeedback, all of which may enhance a patient's sense of personal control and potentially reduce pain. Behavior therapy usually is focused on improving the functional capabilities of the patient with chronic pain (Fordyce et al. 1986). These cognitive and behavioral approaches, combined with intensive physiatric therapies, are the foundation of the multidisciplinary pain management program, which may be the optimal treatment for a subgroup of patients with chronic nonmalignant pain associated with a high level of disability.

Patients with challenging psychological needs are best referred to a mental health care provider, preferably one with experience in the management of chronic pain. Patients who are unwilling or unable to accept a psychiatric referral may still benefit from treatments implemented by another clinician as part of the broader therapeutic strategy. For example, many patients can benefit from instruction in simple cognitive techniques, such as relaxation training or distraction. A graduated exercise program can be implemented through the use of an activity diary maintained by the patient.

Finally, the comprehensive pain assessment may indicate the need for other types of psychological treatment, including individual insight-oriented therapy or family therapy. Again, these approaches may be viewed as part of a multimodality approach, the goals of which encompass both enhanced comfort and improved physical and psychosocial function.

Conclusion

Effective management of chronic pain requires a comprehensive assessment and a therapeutic approach tailored to each patient's unique needs. A variety of treatment strategies may be used. These strategies include many specific therapies in seven broad categories: pharmacological, anesthesiological, surgical, neurostimulatory, physiatric, psychological, and complementary. Optimal management requires ongoing assessment and a willingness to alter the approach as needed.

Pharmacological management involves the use of one or more agents from three major drug classes: nonopioid, adjuvant, and opioid analgesics. The COX-2–specific inhibitors have recently expanded nonopioid treatment options. These drugs are analgesic and anti-inflammatory and have less GI toxicity than the nonselective COX inhibitors. The available adjuvant analgesics continue to expand as pain-relieving properties are attributed to an ever-widening group of drugs. These drugs are particularly useful for pain syndromes, such as neuropathic pain, that are relatively less responsive to traditional analgesics. Opioids are first-line therapy for cancer pain and are playing an increasing role in the management of intractable nonmalignant pain. Unfortunately, their use continues to be limited by fear and misconceptions. Lack of understanding about the distinction between tolerance, physical dependence, and addiction impedes the appropriate use of these drugs.

Anesthesiological, surgical, neurostimulatory, and physiatric therapies can be used alone or in conjunction with pharmacological interventions. For many patients, psychological factors may sustain pain and pain behaviors. Skilled evaluation and intervention by mental health professionals familiar with the treatment of chronic pain is a critical dimension of comprehensive pain management. Coordinating interdisciplinary care and providing appropriate therapies for the patient's pain, disability, and comorbid conditions can be two of the most challenging aspects of chronic pain management.

References

Abram SE, Lightfoot RW: Treatment of long-standing causalgia with prazosin. Regional Anesthesia 6:79–81, 1981

Agency for Health Care Policy and Research Acute Pain Management Panel: Acute Pain Management: Operative or Medical Procedures and Trauma. Washington, DC, U.S. Department of Health and Human Services, 1992

Albe-Fessard D, Lombard MC: Use of an animal model to evaluate the origin of deafferentation pain and protection against it, in Advances in Pain Research and Therapy, Vol 5: Proceedings of the Third World Congress on Pain. Edited by Bonica JJ, Lindblom U, Iggo A. New York, Raven, 1982, pp 691–700

Anthony M, Lance JW: MAO inhibition in the treatment of migraine. Arch Neurol 21:263–268, 1969

Arner S, Rawal N, Gustafsson LL: Clinical experience of long-term treatment with epidural and intrathecal opioids—a nationwide survey, Acta Anaesthesiol Scand 32:253–259, 1988

Backonja M, Beidoun A, Edwards KR, et al: Gabapentin for the symptomatic treatment of painful neuropathy in patients with diabetes mellitus. JAMA 280:1831–1836, 1998

Banning A, Sjogren P: Cerebral effects of long-term oral opioids in cancer patients measured by continuous reaction time. Clin J Pain 6:91–95, 1990

Baranowski AP, De Courcey J, Bonello E: A trial of intravenous lidocaine on the pain and allodynia of postherpetic neuralgia. J Pain Symptom Manage 17:429–433, 1999

Bercel NA: Cyclobenzaprine in the treatment of skeletal muscle spasm in osteoarthritis of the cervical and lumbar spine. Current Therapeutic Research 22:462–468, 1977

Berkley KJ: On the dorsal columns: translating basic research hypotheses to clinic. Pain 70:103–107, 1997

Besson J-M, Chaouch A: Peripheral and spinal mechanisms of nociception. Physiol Rev 67:67–185, 1987

Birkeland IW, Clawson DK: Drug combinations with orphenadrine for pain relief associated with muscle spasm. Clin Pharmacol Ther 9:639–646, 1968

Blom S: Tic douloureux treated with new anticonvulsant. Arch Neurol 9:285–290, 1963

Boas RA, Covino BG, Shaharian A: Analgesic responses to IV lidocaine. Br J Anaesth 54:501–505, 1982

Bonicalzi V, Canavero S, Cerutti F, et al: Lamotrigine reduces total postoperative analgesic requirement: a randomized double-blind, placebo-controlled pilot study. Surgery 122:567–570, 1997

Bowsher D: The effects of pre-emptive treatment of postherpetic neuralgia with amitriptyline: a randomized, double-blind, placebo-controlled trial. J Pain Symptom Manage 13:327–331, 1997

Braham J, Saia A: Phenytoin in the treatment of trigeminal and other neuralgias. Lancet 2:892–893, 1960

Brena SF, Sanders SH: Opioids in nonmalignant pain: questions in search of answers. Clin J Pain 7:342–345, 1991

Brescia FJ, Portenoy RK, Ryan M, et al: Pain, opioid use and survival in hospitalized patients with advanced cancer. J Clin Oncol 10:149–155, 1992

Brodner RA, Taub A: Chronic pain exacerbated by long-term narcotic use in patients with nonmalignant disease: clinical syndrome and treatment. Mt Sinai J Med 45:233–237, 1978

Brose WG, Cousins MJ: Subcutaneous lidocaine for the treatment of neuropathic cancer pain. Pain 45:145–148, 1991

Bruera E, Roca E, Cedaro L, et al: Action of oral methylprednisolone in terminal cancer patients: a prospective randomized double-blind study. Cancer Treatment Reports 69:751–754, 1985

Bruera E, Chadwick S, Brenneis C, et al: Methylphenidate associated with narcotics for the treatment of cancer pain. Cancer Treatment Reports 71:67–70, 1987

Bruera E, Macmillan K, Hanson J, et al: The cognitive effects of the administration of narcotic analgesics in patients with cancer pain. Pain 39:13–16, 1989a

Bruera E, MacMillan D, Hanson J, et al: The Edmonton Staging System for Cancer Pain: preliminary report. Pain 37:203–210, 1989b

Bruera E, Ripamonti C, Brenneis C, et al: A randomized double-blind crossover trial of intravenous lidocaine in the treatment of neuropathic cancer pain. J Pain Symptom Manage 7:138–140, 1992

Buckley FP, Sizemore WA, Charlton JE: Medication management in patients with chronic non-malignant pain: a review of the use of a drug withdrawal protocol. Pain 26:153–166, 1986

Burchiel KJ: Neurosurgical procedures of the peripheral nerves, in Neurosurgical Management of Pain. Edited by North RB, Levy RM. New York, Springer, 1997, pp 133–162

Burnham R, Gregg R, Healy P, et al: The effectiveness of topical diclofenac for lateral epicondylitis. Clin J Sport Med 8:78–81, 1998

Butler S: Present status of tricyclic antidepressants in chronic pain, in Advances in Pain Research and Therapy, Vol 7: Recent Advances in the Management of Pain. Edited by Benedetti CR, Chapman CR, Moricca G. New York, Raven, 1984, pp 173–198

Byas-Smith MG, Max MB, Muir H, et al: Transdermal clonidine compared to placebo in painful diabetic neuropathy using a two-staged "enriched enrollment" design. Pain 60:267–274, 1995

Caccia MR: Clonazepam in facial neuralgia and cluster headache: clinical and electrophysiological study. Eur Neurol 13:560–563, 1975

Campbell FG, Graham JG, Silkha KJ: Clinical trial of carbamazepine (Tegretol) in trigeminal neuralgia. J Neurol Neurosurg Psychiatry 29:265–267, 1966

Cantor FK: Phenytoin treatment of thalamic pain (letter). BMJ 2:590, 1972

Caraceni A, Portenoy RK: Pain management in patients with pancreatic cancer. Cancer 78:639–654, 1996

Caraceni A, Portenoy RK: Pain, in Clinical Neurology. Edited by Griggs RC, Joynt RJ. Philadelphia, PA, Lippincott-Raven (in press)

Caraceni A, Zecca E, Martini C, et al: Gabapentin as adjuvant to opioid analgesia for neuropathic cancer pain. J Pain Symptom Manage 17:441–445, 1999

Cerbo R, Barbanti P, Fabbrini G, et al: Amitriptyline is effective in chronic but not in episodic tension-type headache: pathogenetic implications. Headache 38:453–457, 1998

Chabal C, Jacobson L, Chaney EF, et al: Narcotics for chronic pain: yes or no? a useless dichotomy. American Pain Society Journal 1:276–281, 1992

Chadda VS, Mathur MS: Double blind study of the effects of diphenylhydantoin sodium in diabetic neuropathy. J Assoc Physicians India 26:403–406, 1978

Cherny NI, Thaler HT, Friedlander-Klar H, et al: Opioid responsiveness of cancer pain syndromes caused by neuropathic or nociceptive mechanisms: a combined analysis of controlled single dose studies. Neurology 44:857–861, 1994

Cheshire WP: Felbamate relieved trigeminal neuralgia. Clin J Pain 11:139–142, 1995

Cleeland CS, Gonin R, Hatfield AK, et al: Pain and its treatment in outpatients with metastatic cancer. N Engl J Med 330:592–597, 1994

Cochin J, Kornetsky C: Development and loss of tolerance to morphine in the rat after single and multiple injections. J Pharmacol Exp Ther 145:1–20, 1964

Couch JR, Ziegler DK, Hassanein R: Amitriptyline in the prophylaxis of migraine effectiveness and relationship of antimigraine and antidepressant effects. Neurology 26:121–127, 1976

Cousins MJ, Cherry DA, Gourlay GK: Acute and chronic pain: use of spinal opioids, in Neural Blockade in Clinical Anesthesia and Management of Pain. Edited by Cousins MJ, Bridenbaugh PO. Philadelphia, PA, JB Lippincott, 1988a, pp 955–1029

Cousins MJ, Dwyer B, Gibb D: Chronic pain and neurolytic blockade, in Neural Blockade in Clinical Anesthesia and Management of Pain. Edited by Cousins MJ, Bridenbaugh PO. Philadelphia, PA, JB Lippincott, 1988b, pp 1053–1084

Dalsgaard J, Flesby S, Juelsgaard P, et al: Low-dose intra-articular morphine analgesia in day-care knee arthroscopy: a randomized, double-blinded, prospective study. Pain 56:151–154, 1994

Davidoff G, Guarracini M, Roth E, et al: Trazodone hydrochloride in the treatment of dysesthetic pain in traumatic myelopathy: a randomized, double-blind, placebo-controlled study. Pain 29:151–161, 1987

Dejgard A, Petersen P, Kastrup J: Mexiletine for treatment of chronic painful diabetic neuropathy. Lancet 1:9–11, 1988

de Leon Casasola OA, Kent E, Lema MJ: Neurolytic superior hypogastric plexus block for chronic pelvic pain associated with cancer. Pain 54:145–151, 1993

Della Cuna GR, Pellegrini A, Piazzi M: Effect of methylprednisolone sodium succinate on quality of life in preterminal cancer patients: a placebo-controlled multicenter study. Eur J Cancer 25:1817–1821, 1989

Derby S, Chin J, Portenoy RK: Systemic opioid therapy for chronic cancer pain: practical guidelines for converting drugs and routes of administration. CNS Drugs 9(2):99–109, 1998

Devor M: The pathophysiology of damaged peripheral nerves, in Textbook of Pain, 3rd Edition. Edited by Wall PD, Melzack R. Edinburgh, Churchill Livingstone, 1994, pp 79–100

Dickenson AH: Where and how do opioids act?, in Progress in Pain Research and Management, Vol 2: Proceedings of the 7th World Congress on Pain. Edited by Gebhart GF, Hammond DL, Jensen TS. Seattle, WA, IASP Press, 1994, pp 525–552

Donohoe RM, Falek A: Neuroimmunomodulation by opiates and other drugs of abuse: relationship to HIV infection and AIDS. Adv Biochem Psychopharmacol 44:145–158, 1988

Drewes AM, Andreasen A, Poulsen LH: Valproate for treatment of chronic central pain after spinal cord injury: a double-blind cross-over study. Paraplegia 32:565–569, 1994

Du Pen SL, Kharasch ED, Williams A, et al: Chronic epidural bupivacaine-opioid infusion in intractable cancer pain. Pain 49:293–300, 1992

Eberhard G, von Knorring L, Nilsson HL, et al: A double-blind randomized study of clomipramine versus maprotiline in patients with idiopathic pain syndromes. Neuropsychobiology 19:25–34, 1988

Ehrenstrom GME, Reiz SLA: EMLA—a eutectic mixture of local anesthetics for topical anesthesia. Acta Anaesthesiol Scand 26:596–598, 1982

Eisenach JC, Du Pen S, Dubois M, et al: The Epidural Clonidine Study Group: epidural clonidine analgesia for intractable cancer pain. Pain 61:391–399, 1995

Ekbom K: Carbamazepine in the treatment of tabetic lightning pains. Arch Neurol 26:374–378, 1972

Ellemann K, Sjogren P, Banning AM, et al: Trial of intravenous lidocaine on painful neuropathy in cancer patients. Clin J Pain 5:291–294, 1989

Elliot F, Little A, Milbrandt W: Carbamazepine for phantom limb phenomena (letter). N Engl J Med 295:678, 1976

Espir MLE, Millac P: Treatment of paroxysmal disorders in multiple sclerosis with carbamazepine (Tegretol). J Neurol Neurosurg Psychiatry 33:528–531, 1970

Evans W, Gensler F, Blackwell B, et al: The effects of antidepressant drugs on pain relief and mood in the chronically ill. Psychosomatics 14:214–219, 1973

Fernandez F, Adams F, Holmes VF: Analgesic effect of alprazolam in patients with chronic organic pain of malignant origin. J Clin Psychopharmacol 7:167–169, 1987

Ferrante FM, Bedder M, Caplan RA, et al: Practice guidelines for cancer pain management: a report by the American Society of Anesthesiologists Task Force on Pain Management, Cancer Pain Section. Anesthesiology 84:1243–1257, 1996a

Ferrante FM, Paggioli J, Cherukuri S, et al: The analgesic response to intravenous lidocaine in the treatment of neuropathic pain. Anesth Analg 82:91–97, 1996b

Field MJ, Oles RJ, Lewis AS, et al: Gabapentin (Neurontin) and S-(+)-3-isobutylgaba represent a novel class of selective antihyperalgesic agents. Br J Pharmacol 121:1513–1522, 1997

Finlayson RD, Maruta T, Morse BR: Substance dependence and chronic pain: profile of 50 patients treated in an alcohol and drug dependence unit. Pain 26:167–174, 1986a

Finlayson RD, Maruta T, Morse BR, et al: Substance dependence and chronic pain: experience with treatment and follow-up results. Pain 26:175–180, 1986b

Fishbain DA, Rosomoff HL, Rosomoff RS: Drug abuse, dependence, and addiction in chronic pain patients. Clin J Pain 8:77–85, 1992

Foley KM: Changing concepts of tolerance to opioids: what the cancer patient has taught us, in Current and Emerging Issues in Cancer Pain: Research and Practice. Edited by Chapman CR, Foley KM. New York, Raven, 1993, pp 331–350

Fordyce WE, Brockway J, Bergman J, et al: A control group comparison of behavioral versus traditional management methods of acute back pain. J Behav Med 9:127–140, 1986

Forrest WH, Brown B, Brown C, et al: Dextroamphetamine with morphine for the treatment of postoperative pain. N Engl J Med 296:712–715, 1977

France RD, Urban BJ, Keefe FJ: Long-term use of narcotic analgesics in chronic pain. Soc Sci Med 19:1379–1382, 1984

Fromm GH, Terence CF, Chatta AS: Baclofen in the treatment of trigeminal neuralgia. Ann Neurol 15:240–247, 1984

Galer BS, Miller KV, Rowbotham MC: Response to intravenous lidocaine differs based on clinical diagnosis and site of nervous system injury. Neurology 43:1233–1235, 1993

Gatchel RJ, Turk DC: Psychological Approaches to Pain Management. New York, Guilford, 1996

Gee NS, Brown JP, Dissanayake VU, et al: The novel anticonvulsant drug, gabapentin (Neurontin), binds to the alpha2delta subunit of a calcium channel. J Biol Chem 271:5768–5776, 1996

Gersh MR, Wolf SL: Application of transcutaneous elective nerve stimulation in the management of patients with pain: state-of-the-art update. Phys Ther 65:314–336, 1985

Gestin Y, Vainio A, Pegurier AM: Long-term intrathecal infusion of morphine in the home care of patients with advanced cancer. Acta Anaesthesiol Scand 41:12–16, 1997

Getto CJ, Sorkness CA, Howell T: Antidepressants and chronic nonmalignant pain: a review. J Pain Symptom Manage 2:9–18, 1987

Ghostine SY, Comair YG, Turner DM, et al: Phenoxybenzamine in the treatment of causalgia. J Neurosurg 60:1263–1268, 1984

Gingras MA: A clinical trial of Tofranil in rheumatic pain in general practice. J Int Med Res 4:41–49, 1976

Gobelet C, Waldburger M, Meier JL: The effect of adding calcitonin to physical treatment on reflex sympathetic dystrophy. Pain 48:171–175, 1992

Gold RH: Treatment of low back syndrome with oral orphenadrine citrate. Current Therapeutic Research 23:271–276, 1978

Goldenberg D, Mayskiy M, Mossey C, et al: A randomized, double-blind crossover trial of fluoxetine and amitriptyline in the treatment of fibromyalgia. Arthritis Rheum 39:1852–1859, 1996

Goldlust A, Su TZ, Welty DF, et al: Effects of anticonvulsant drug gabapentin on the enzymes in metabolic pathways of glutamate and GABA. Epilepsy Res 22:1–11, 1995

Gonzales GR, Elliott KJ, Portenoy RK, et al: The impact of a comprehensive evaluation in the management of cancer pain. Pain 47:141–144, 1991

Goodkin K, Gullion CM, Agras WS: A randomized, double blind, placebo-controlled trial of trazodone hydrochloride in chronic low back pain syndrome. J Clin Psychopharmacol 10:269–278, 1990

Gourlay GK, Cherry DA: Can opioids be successfully used to treat severe pain in nonmalignant conditions? Clin J Pain 7:347–349, 1991

Green JB: Dilantin in the treatment of lightning pains. Neurology 11:257–258, 1961

Gybels J: Commisural myelotomy revisited (editorial). Pain 70:1–2, 1997

Haertzen CA, Hooks NT: Changes in personality and subjective experience associated with the chronic administration and withdrawal of opiates. J Nerv Ment Dis 148:606–614, 1969

Hameroff SR, Cork RC, Scherer K, et al: Doxepin effects on chronic pain, depression and plasma opioids. J Clin Psychiatry 43:22–27, 1982

Hammond DL: Pharmacology of central pain-modulating networks (biogenic amines and nonopioid analgesics), in Advances in Pain Research and Therapy, Vol 9: Proceedings of the Fourth World Congress on Pain. Edited by Fields HL, Dubner R, Cervero F. New York, Raven, 1985, pp 499–513

Hanks GW, Trueman T, Twycross RG: Corticosteroids in terminal cancer. Postgrad Med J 59:702–706, 1983

Hatangdi VS, Boas RA, Richards EG: Postherpetic neuralgia: management with antiepileptic and tricyclic drugs, in Advances in Pain Research and Therapy, Vol 1. Edited by Bonica JJ, Albe-Fessard D. New York, Raven, 1976, pp 583–587

Hendler N, Cimini C, Ma T, et al: A comparison of cognitive impairment due to benzodiazepines and to narcotics. Am J Psychiatry 137:828–830, 1980

Hirata K, Koyama N, Minami T: The effects of clonidine and itzanidine on responses of nociceptive neurons in nucleus ventralis posterolateralis of the cat thalamus. Anesth Analg 81(2):259–264, 1995

Hogan Q, Haddox JD, Abram S, et al: Epidural opiates and local anesthetics for the management of cancer pain. Pain 46:271–279, 1991

Hoskin PJ, Hanks GW: Opioid agonist-antagonist drugs in acute and chronic pain states. Drugs 41:326–344, 1991

Houde RW: Nathan B. Eddy Memorial Lecture: the analgesic connection, in: Problems of Drug Dependence (NIDA Res Monogr 55). Edited by Harris LS. Rockville, MD, National Institute on Drug Abuse, 1985, pp 4–13

Houde RW, Wallenstein SL, Beaver WT: Evaluation of analgesics in patients with cancer pain, in International Encyclopedia of Pharmacology and Therapeutics, Section 6, Vol 1: Clinical Pharmacology. Edited by Lasagna L. Oxford, England, Pergamon, 1966, pp 59–98

Ischia S, Ischia A, Luzzani A, et al: Results up to death in the treatment of persistent cervico-thoracic (Pancoast) and thoracic malignant pain by unilateral percutaneous cervical cordotomy. Pain 21:339–355, 1985

Jacox A, Carr DB, Payne R, et al: Clinical Practice Guideline Number 9: Management of Cancer Pain (AHCPR Publ No 94-0592). Rockville, MD, U.S. Department of Health and Human Services, Agency for Health Care Policy and Research, 1994

Jadad AR, Carroll D, Glynn CJ, et al: Morphine responsiveness of chronic pain: double-blind randomised crossover study with patient-controlled analgesia. Lancet 339:1367–1371, 1992

Jadad AR, Carroll D, Glynn CJ, et al: Intravenous regional sympathetic blockade for pain relief in reflex sympathetic dystrophy: a systematic review of the literature and a randomized double-blind crossover study. J Pain Symptom Manage 10:13–20, 1995

Jaeger H, Maier C: Calcitonin in phantom limb pain: a double blind study. Pain 48:21–27, 1992

Jaffe JH: Drug addiction and drug abuse, in The Pharmacological Basis of Therapeutics, 7th Edition. Edited by Gilman AG, Goodman LS, Rall TW, et al. New York, Macmillan, 1985, pp 532–581

Jain S, Patt RB: Complications of invasive procedures, in Cancer Pain. Edited by Patt RB. Philadelphia, PA, JB Lippincott, 1993, pp 443–460

Jensen R, Brinck T, Olesen J: Sodium valproate has a prophylactic effect in migraine without aura: a triple-blind, placebo-controlled crossover study. Neurology 44:647–651, 1994

Johansson F, Von Knorring L: A double-blind controlled study of serotonin uptake inhibitor (zimelidine) versus placebo in chronic pain patients. Pain 7:69–78, 1979

Joshi GP, McCarroll SM, O'Brien TM, et al: Intraarticular analgesia following knee arthroscopy. Anesth Analg 76:333–336, 1993

Kaiko RF, Foley KM, Grabinski PY, et al: Central nervous system excitatory effects of meperidine in cancer patients. Ann Neurol 13:180–185, 1983

Kalso E, Tiina T, Pertti NJ: Amitriptyline effectively relieves neuropathic pain following treatment of breast cancer. Pain 64:293–302, 1996

Kanner RM, Foley KM: Patterns of narcotic drug use in a cancer pain clinic. Ann N Y Acad Sci 362:161–172, 1981

Killian JM, Fromm GH: Carbamazepine in the treatment of neuralgia: use and side effects. Arch Neurol 19:129–136, 1968

Kishore-Kumar R, Max MB, Schafer SC, et al: Desipramine relieves postherpetic neuralgia. Clin Pharmacol Ther 47:305–312, 1990

Koesis JD, Honmou O: Gabapentin increases GABA-induced depolarization in rat neonatal optic nerve. Neurosci Lett 169(1-2):181–184, 1994

Kozin F, Ryan LM, Carerra GF, et al: The reflex sympathetic dystrophy syndrome (RSDS). III: scintigraphic studies, further evidence for the therapeutic efficacy of systemic corticosteroids, and proposed diagnostic criteria. Am J Med 70:23–29, 1981

Kreek MJ: Medical complications in methadone patients. Ann N Y Acad Sci 311:110–134, 1978

Kreek MJ, Dodes S, Kane S, et al: Long-term methadone maintenance therapy: effects on liver function. Ann Intern Med 77:598–602, 1972

Kvinsdahl B, Molin J, Froland A, et al: Imipramine treatment of painful diabetic neuropathy. JAMA 251:1727–1730, 1984

Langemark M, Olesen J: Sulpiride and paroxetine in the treatment of chronic tension-type headache: an explanatory double-blind trial. Headache 34:20–24, 1994

Langman MJS, Weil J, Wainwright P, et al: Risks of bleeding peptic ulcer associated with individual nonsteroidal anti-inflammatory drugs. Lancet 343:1075–1078, 1994

Langohr HD, Stohr M, Petruch F: An open and double-blind cross-over study on the efficacy of clomipramine (Anafranil) in patients with painful mono- and polyneuropathies. Eur Neurol 21:309–317, 1982

Lascelles RG: Atypical facial pain and depression. Br J Psychiatry 122:651–659, 1966

Laska EM, Sunshine A, Mueller F, et al: Caffeine as an analgesic adjuvant. JAMA 251:1711–1718, 1984

Lechin F, van der Dijs B, Lechin ME, et al: Pimozide therapy for trigeminal neuralgia. Arch Neurol 9:960–962, 1989

Lindstrom P, Lindblom U: The analgesic effect of tocainide in trigeminal neuralgia. Pain 28:45–50, 1987

Lipton S: Neurodestructive procedures in the management of cancer pain. J Pain Symptom Manage 4:219–228, 1987

Lockman LA, Hunninghake DB, Drivit W, et al: Relief of pain of Fabry's disease by dephenylhydantoin. Neurology 23:871–875, 1973

Loeb DS, Ahlquist DA, Talley NJ: Management of gastroduodenopathy associated with use of nonsteroidal anti-inflammatory drugs. Mayo Clin Proc 67:354–364, 1992

Loeser JD, Ward AA, White LE: Chronic deafferentation of human spinal cord neurons. J Neurosurg 29:48–50, 1968

Lombardo WK, Lombardo B, Goldstein A: Cognitive functioning under moderate and low dose methadone maintenance. International Journal of the Addictions 11:389–401, 1976

Mao J, Price DD, Mayer DJ: Mechanisms of hyperalgesia and morphine tolerance: a current view of their possible interaction. Pain 62:259–274, 1995

Mao J, Price DD, Caruso FS, et al: Oral administration of dextromethorphan prevents the development of morphine tolerance and dependence in rats. Pain 67:361–368, 1996

Marchettini P, Lacerenza M, Marangoni C, et al: Lidocaine test in neuralgia. Pain 48:377–382, 1992

Martin G: The management of pain following laminectomy for lumbar disc lesions. Ann R Coll Surg Engl 63:244–252, 1981

Mathisen LC, Skjelbred P, Skoglund LA, et al: Effect of ketamine, an NMDA receptor inhibitor, in acute and chronic orofacial pain. Pain 61:215–220, 1995

Max MB, Gilron I: Sympathetically-maintained pain: has the emperor no clothes ? Neurology 52:905–907, 1999

Max MB, Culnane M, Schafer SC, et al: Amitriptyline relieves diabetic neuropathy pain in patients with normal or depressed mood. Neurology 37:589–594, 1987

Max MB, Kishore-Kumar R, Schafer SC, et al: Efficacy of desipramine in painful diabetic neuropathy: a placebo-controlled trial. Pain 45:3–9, 1991

Max MB, Lynch SA, Muir J, et al: Effects of desipramine, amitriptyline, and fluoxetine on pain in diabetic neuropathy. N Engl J Med 326:1250–1256, 1992

McCormack K, Brune K: Dissociation between the antinociceptive and anti-inflammatory effects of the non-steroidal anti-inflammatory drugs. Drugs 41:533–547, 1991

McGraw T, Koseck P: Erythromelalgia pain managed with gabapentin. Anesthesiology 86:988–990, 1997

McNairy SL, Maruta T, Ivnik RJ, et al: Prescription medication dependence and neuropsychologic function. Pain 18:169–177, 1984

McQuay H, Moore A: An Evidence-Based Resource for Pain Relief. Oxford, England, Oxford University Press, 1998

McQuay HJ, Jadad AR, Carroll D, et al: Opioid sensitivity of chronic pain: a patient-controlled analgesia method. Anaesthesia 47:757–767, 1992

McQuay HJ, Carroll D, Jadad AR, et al: Dextromethorphan for the treatment of neuropathic pain: a double-blind randomised controlled crossover trial with integral n-1 design. Pain 59:127–133, 1994

Medina JL, Diamond S: Drug dependency in patients with chronic headache. Headache 17:12–14, 1977

Mellick GA, Mellick LB: Reflex sympathetic dystrophy treated with gabapentin. Arch Phys Med Rehabil 78:98–105, 1997

Mercadante S: Pain treatment and outcomes for patients with advanced cancer who receive follow-up care at home. Cancer 85:1849–1858, 1999

Mercadante S, Maddaloni S, Roccella S, et al: Predictive factors in advanced cancer pain treated only by analgesics. Pain 50:151–155, 1992

Mercadante S, Lodi F, Sapio M, et al: Long-term ketamine subcutaneous continuous infusion in neuropathic cancer pain. J Pain Symptom Manage 10:564–568, 1995

Mercadante S, Sapio M, Caligara M, et al: Opioid sparing effect of diclofenac in cancer pain. J Pain Symptom Manage 14:15–20, 1997

Mercadante S, Casuccio A, Genovese G: Ineffectiveness of dextromethorphan in cancer pain. J Pain Symptom Manage 16:317–322, 1998

Merry AF, Schug SA, Richards EG, et al: Opioids in chronic pain of nonmalignant origin: state of the debate in New Zealand. European Journal of Pain 13:39–43, 1992

Miller R, Eisenkraft JB, Cohen M, et al: Midazolam as an adjunct to meperidine analgesia for postoperative pain. Clin J Pain 2:37–43, 1986

Molitor TW, Morilla A, Risdahl JM, et al: Chronic morphine administration impairs cell-mediated immune responses in swine. J Pharmacol Exp Ther 260:581–586, 1992

Moulin DE, Iezzi A, Amireh R, et al: Randomised trial of oral morphine for chronic noncancer pain. Lancet 347:143–147, 1996

Mullan S: Surgical management of pain in cancer of the head and neck. Surg Clin North Am 53:203–210, 1973

Murray MD, Brater DC: Renal toxicity of the nonsteroidal anti-inflammatory drugs. Annu Rev Pharmacol Toxicol 33:435–465, 1993

Nashold BS, Ostdahl RH: Dorsal root entry zone lesions for pain relief. J Neurosurg 51:59–69, 1979

Nelson KA, Park KM, Robinovitz E, et al: High-dose oral dextromethorphan versus placebo in painful diabetic neuropathy and post-herpetic neuralgia. Neurology 48:1212–1218, 1997

North RB, Kidd DH, Zahurak M, et al: Spinal cord stimulation for chronic, intractable pain: experience over two decades. Neurosurgery 32:384–394, 1993

Numo R: Prevention of NSAID-induced ulcers by the co-administration of misoprostol: implications in clinical practice. Scand J Rheumatol 92 (suppl):25–29, 1992

Nystrom B, Hagbarth KE: Microelectrode recordings from transected nerves in amputees in phantom limb pain. Neurosci Lett 27:211–216, 1981

Ochshorn M, Novick DM, Kreek MJ: In vitro studies of the effect of methadone on natural killer cell activity. Isr J Med Sci 26:421–425, 1990

Okasha A, Ghaleb AA, Sadek A: A double-blind trial for the clinical management of psychogenic headache. Br J Psychiatry 122:181–183, 1973

Passik SD, Portenoy RK: Substance abuse issues in palliative care, in Supportive Oncology. Edited by Berger A, Levy M, Portenoy RK, et al. New York, JB Lippincott, 1998, pp 513–530

Peiris JB, Perera GLS, Devendra SV, et al: Sodium valproate in trigeminal neuralgia (letter). Med J Aust 2:278, 1980

Perry S, Heidrich G: Management of pain during debridement: a survey of U.S. burn units. Pain 13:267–280, 1982

Persson J, Axelsson G, Hallin RG, et al: Beneficial effects of ketamine in a chronic pain state with allodynia, possibly due to central sensitization. Pain 60:217–222, 1995

Pilowsky I, Hallet EC, Bassett KL, et al: A controlled study of amitriptyline in the treatment of chronic pain. Pain 14:169–179, 1982

Plummer JL, Cherry DA, Cousins MJ, et al: Long-term spinal administration of morphine in cancer and non-cancer pain: a retrospective study. Pain 44:215–220, 1991

Portenoy RK: Pharmacologic management of chronic pain, in Pain Syndromes in Neurology. Edited by Fields HL. London, Butterworths, 1990, pp 257–278

Portenoy RK: Opioid therapy for chronic nonmalignant pain: current status, in Progress in Pain Research and Management, Vol 1: Pharmacological Approaches to the Treatment of Chronic Pain: New Concepts and Critical Issues. Edited by Fields HL, Liebeskind JC. Seattle, WA, IASP Press, 1994a, pp 247–288

Portenoy RK: Opioid tolerance and responsiveness: research findings and clinical observations, in Progress in Pain Research and Management, Vol 2: Proceedings of the 7th World Congress on Pain. Edited by Gebhart GF, Hammond DL, Jensen TS. Seattle, WA, IASP Press, 1994b, pp 595–619

Portenoy RK: Contemporary Diagnosis and Management of Pain in Oncologic and AIDS Patients, 2nd Edition. Newtown, PA, Handbooks in Healthcare, 1998

Portenoy RK, Cheville AL: Chronic pain management, in Psychiatric Care of the Medical Patient, 2nd Edition. Edited by Stoudemire A, Fogel BS, Greenberg DB. New York, Oxford University Press, 2000, pp 199–225

Portenoy RK, Foley KM: Chronic use of opioid analgesics in non-malignant pain: report of 38 cases. Pain 25:171–186, 1986

Portenoy RK, Payne R: Acute and chronic pain, in Substance Abuse: A Comprehensive Textbook, 3rd Edition. Edited by Lowinson JH, Ruiz P, Millman RB, et al. Baltimore, MD, Williams & Wilkins, 1997, pp 563–590

Portenoy RK, Foley KM, Inturrisi CE: The nature of opioid responsiveness and its implications for neuropathic pain: new hypotheses derived from studies of opioid infusions. Pain 43:273–286, 1990

Porter J, Jick H: Addiction rare in patients treated with narcotics (letter). N Engl J Med 302:123, 1980

Power-Smith P, Turkington D: Fluoxetine in phantom limb pain. Br J Psychiatry 163:105–106, 1993

Pranikoff K, Constantino G: The use of amitriptyline in patients with urinary frequency and pain. Urology 51(suppl 5A):179–181, 1998

Price DD, Mao J, Frenk H, et al: The N-methyl-d-apartate receptor antagonist dextomethorphan selectively reduces temporal summation of second pain in man. Pain 59:165–174, 1994

Price DD, Mao J, Lu J, et al: Effects of the combined oral administration of NSAIDs and dextromethorphan on behavioral symptoms indicative of arthritic pain in rats. Pain 68:119–127, 1996

Prough DS, McLeskey CH, Borshy GG, et al: Efficacy of oral nifedipine in the treatment of reflex sympathetic dystrophy. Anesthesiology 62:796–799, 1985

Raftery H: The management of postherpetic pain using sodium valproate and amitriptyline. Journal of the Irish Medical Association 72:399–401, 1979

Rall TW, Schleifer LS: Drugs effective in the therapy of the epilepsies, in The Pharmacological Basis of Therapeutics, 7th Edition. Edited by Gilman AG, Goodman LS, Rall TW, et al. New York, Macmillan, 1985, pp 446–472

Rani PU, Naidu MU, Prasad VB, et al: An evaluation of antidepressants in rheumatic pain conditions. Anesth Analg 83:371–375, 1996

Raskin NH, Levinson SA, Hoffman PM, et al: Postsympathectomy neuralgia: amelioration with diphenylhydantoin and carbamazepine. Am J Surg 128:75–78, 1974

Rinaldi RC, Steindler EM, Wilford BB, et al: Clarification and standardization of substance abuse terminology. JAMA 259:555–557, 1988

Rockliff BW, Davis EH: Controlled sequential trials of carbamazepine in trigeminal neuralgia. Arch Neurol 15:129–136, 1966

Rosenberg JM, Harrell C, Ristic H, et al: The effect of gabapentin on neuropathic pain. Clin J Pain 13:251–255, 1997

Rothrock JF: Clinical studies of valproate for migraine prophylaxis. Cephalalgia 17:81–83, 1997

Rowbotham MC: Topical analgesic agents, in Pharmacological Approaches to the Treatment of Chronic Pain: New Concepts and Critical Issues. Edited by Fields HL, Liebeskind JC. Seattle, WA, IASP Press, 1994, pp 211–227

Rowbotham MC, Reisner L, Fields HL: Both intravenous lidocaine and morphine reduce the pain of postherpetic neuralgia. Neurology 41:102–104, 1991

Rowbotham MC, Davies PS, Fields HL: Topical lidocaine gel relieves postherpetic neuralgia. Ann Neurol 37:246–253, 1995

Rowbotham M, Harden N, Stacey B, et al: Gabapentin for the treatment of postherpetic neuralgia. JAMA 280:1837–1842, 1998

Rull JA, Quibrera R, Gonzalez-Milan H, et al: Symptomatic treatment of peripheral diabetic neuropathy with carbamazepine (Tegretol): double blind cross-over trial. Diabetologia 5:215–218, 1969

Rumore MM, Schlichting DA: Clinical efficacy of antihistamines as analgesics. Pain 25:7–22, 1986

Samkoff LM, Daras M, Tuchman AJ, et al: Amelioration of refractory dysesthetic limb pain in multiple sclerosis by gabapentin. Neurology 49:304–305, 1997

Sanders M, Zurmond W: Safety of unilateral and bilateral percutaneous cordotomy in 80 terminally ill cancer patients. J Clin Oncol 13:1509–1512, 1995

Sandford PR, Lindblom LB, Haddox JD: Amitriptyline and carbamazepine in the treatment of dysesthetic pain in spinal cord injury. Arch Phys Med Rehabil 73:300–301, 1992

Saper JR, Silberstein SD, Lake AE, et al: Double-blind trial of fluoxetine: chronic daily headache and migraine. Headache 34:497–502, 1994

Schmid RL, Sanler AN, Katz J: Use and efficacy of low-dose ketamine in the management of acute postoperative pain: a review of current techniques and outcome. Pain 82:111–125, 1999

Schofferman J: Long-term use of opioid analgesics for the treatment of chronic pain of nonmalignant origin. J Pain Symptom Manage 8:279–288, 1993

Schott GD: Visceral afferents: their contribution to "sympathetic dependent" pain. Brain 117:397–413, 1994

Schubert TT, Bologna SD, Nensey Y, et al: Ulcer risk factors: interactions between Helicobacter pylori infection, nonsteroidal use, and age. Am J Med 94:413–418, 1993

Schug SA, Zech D, Dorr U: Cancer pain management according to WHO analgesic guidelines. J Pain Symptom Manage 5:27–32, 1990

Schug SA, Zech D, Grond S, et al: A long-term survey of morphine in cancer pain patients. J Pain Symptom Manage 7:259–266, 1992

Segal AZ, Rordorf G: Gabapentin as a novel treatment for postherpetic neuralgia. Neurology 46:1175–1176, 1996

Shavit Y, Lewis JW, Terman WG, et al: Opioid peptides mediate the suppressive effect of stress on natural killer cell cytotoxicity. Science 223:188–190, 1984

Shavit Y, Martin FC, Yirmiya R, et al: Effects of a single administration of morphine or footshock on natural killer cell cytotoxicity. Brain Behav Immun 1:318–328, 1987

Silberstein SD: Divalproex sodium in headache: literature review and clinical guidelines. Headache 36:547–555, 1996

Simon LS: Nonsteroidal anti-inflammatory drug toxicity. Curr Opin Rheumatol 5:265–275, 1993

Simson G: Propranolol for causalgia and Sudek's atrophy (letter). JAMA 227:327, 1974

Sindrup SH, Gram LF, Brosen K, et al: The selective serotonin reuptake inhibitor paroxetine is effective in the treatment of diabetic neuropathy symptoms. Pain 42:135–144, 1990

Sindrup SH, Bjerre U, Dejgaard A, et al: The selective serotonin reuptake inhibitor citalopram relieves the symptoms of diabetic neuropathy. Clin Pharmacol Ther 52:547–552, 1992

Singh PN, Sharma P, Gupta PK, et al: Clinical evaluation of diazepam for relief of postoperative pain. Br J Anaesth 53:831–836, 1981

Sist TC, Filadora VA, Miner M, et al: Experience with gabapentin for neuropathic pain in the head and neck: report of ten cases. Regional Anesthesia 22:473–478, 1997a

Sist T, Filadora V, Miner M, et al: Gabapentin for idiopathic trigeminal neuralgia: report of two cases (letter). Neurology 48:1467, 1997b

Sjoberg M, Appelgren L, Einarsson S, et al: Long-term intrathecal morphine and bupivacaine in "refractory" cancer pain: results from the first series of 52 patients. Acta Anaesthesiol Scand 35:30–43, 1991

Sjogren P, Banning A: Pain, sedation and reaction time during long-term treatment of cancer patients with oral and epidural opioids. Pain 39:5–12, 1989

Smith CM: Relaxants of skeletal muscle, in Physiological Pharmacology, Vol 2. Edited by Root WS, Hoffmann FG. New York, Academic Press, 1966, pp 2–96

Spiegel K, Kalb R, Pasternak GW: Analgesic activity of tricyclic antidepressants. Ann Neurol 13:462–465, 1983

Stambaugh JE, Lance C: Analgesic efficacy and pharmacokinetic evaluation of meperidine and hydroxyzine, alone and in combination. Cancer Invest 1:111–117, 1983

Stein C: Interaction of immune-competent cells and nociceptors, in Progress in Pain Research and Management, Vol 2: Proceedings of the 7th World Congress on Pain. Edited by Gebhart GF, Hammond DL, Jensen TS. Seattle, WA, IASP Press, 1994, pp 285–297

Stein C, Hassan AHS, Lehrberger K, et al: Local analgesic effect of endogenous opioid peptides. Lancet 342:321–324, 1993

Steiner TJ, Rindley LJ, Yuen AW: Lamotrigine versus placebo in the prophylaxis of migraine with and without aura. Cephalalgia 17:109–112, 1997

Swanson G, Smith J, Bulich R, et al: Patient-controlled analgesia for chronic cancer pain in the ambulatory setting: a report of 117 patients. J Clin Oncol 7:1903–1908, 1989

Swerdlow M: Anticonvulsant drugs and chronic pain. Clin Neuropharmacol 7:51–82, 1984

Swerdlow M, Cundill JG: Anticonvulsant drugs used in the treatment of lancinating pains: a comparison. Anesthesia 36:1129–1132, 1981

Tabira T, Shibasaki H, Kuroiwa Y: Reflex sympathetic dystrophy (causalgia) treatment with guanethidine. Arch Neurol 40:430–432, 1983

Taha AS, Hudson N, Hawkey CJ, et al: Famotidine for the prevention of gastric and duodenal ulcers caused by nonsteroidal anti-inflammatory drugs. N Engl J Med 334:1435–1439, 1996

Takeda F: Results of field testing in Japan of the WHO Draft Interim Guidelines on Relief of Cancer Pain. Pain Clinic 1:83–89, 1986

Tandan R, Lewis GA, Drusinske PB, et al: Topical capsaicin in painful diabetic neuropathy: controlled study with long-term follow-up. Diabetes Care 15:8–14, 1992

Tanelian DL, Cousins MJ: Combined neurogenic and nociceptive pain in a patient with Pancoast tumor managed by epidural hydromorphone and oral carbamazepine. Pain 36:85–88, 1989

Tannock I, Gospodarowicz M, Meakin W, et al: Treatment of metastatic prostatic cancer with low-dose prednisone: evaluation of pain and quality of life as pragmatic indices of response. J Clin Oncol 7:590–597, 1989

Tasker RR, North R: Cordotomy and myelotomy, in Neurosurgical Management of Pain. Edited by North RB, Levy RM. New York, Springer, 1997, pp 191–220

Taylor PH, Gray K, Bicknell RG, et al: Glossopharyngeal neuralgia with syncope. J Laryngol Otol 91:859–868, 1977

Ter Riet G, Kleijnen J, Knipschild P: Acupuncture and chronic pain: a criteria-based meta-analysis. J Clin Epidemiol 43:1191–1199, 1990

Theesan KA, Marsh WR: Relief of diabetic neuropathy with fluoxetine. DICP 23:572–574, 1989

Turk DC, Meichenbaum D, Genest M: Pain and Behavioral Medicine: A Cognitive-Behavioral Perspective. New York, Guilford, 1983

Vainio A, Ollila J, Matikainen E, et al: Driving ability in cancer patients receiving long-term morphine analgesia. Lancet 346:667–670, 1995

Ventafridda V: Continuing care: a major issue in cancer pain management. Pain 36:137–143, 1989

Ventafridda V, Martino G: Clinical evaluation of subarachnoid neurolytic blocks in intractable cancer pain, in Advances in Pain Research and Therapy, Vol 1. Edited by Bonica JJ, Albe-Fessard D. New York, Raven, 1976, pp 600–703

Ventafridda V, Fochi C, Sganzerla E, et al: Neurolytic blocks in perineal pain, in Advances in Pain Research and Therapy, Vol 2. Edited by Bonica JJ, Ventafridda V. New York, Raven, 1979, pp 597–605

Ventafridda V, Bonezzi C, Caraceni A, et al: Antidepressants for cancer pain and other painful syndromes with deafferentation component: comparison of amitriptyline and trazodone. Ital J Neurol Sci 8:579–587, 1987a

Ventafridda V, Tamburini M, Caraceni A, et al: A validation study of the WHO method for cancer pain relief. Cancer 59:850–856, 1987b

Vrethem M, Boivie J, Arnqvist H, et al: A comparison of amitriptyline and maprotiline in the treatment of painful polyneuropathy in diabetics and nondiabetics. Clin J Pain 13:313–323, 1997

Waldman SD: Implantable drug delivery systems: practical considerations. J Pain Symptom Manage 5:169–175, 1990

Waldman SD, Coombs DW: Selection of implantable narcotic delivery systems. Anesth Analg 68:377–384, 1989

Waldman SD, Leak DW, Kennedy LD, et al: Intraspinal opioid therapy, in Cancer Pain. Edited by Patt RB. Philadelphia, PA, JB Lippincott, 1993, pp 285–328

Wall PD, Gutnick M: Ongoing activity in peripheral nerves, 2: the physiology and pharmacology of impulses originating in a neuroma. Exp Neurol 43:580–593, 1974

Ward SE, Goldberg N, Miller-McCauley V, et al: Patient-related barriers to management of cancer pain. Pain 52:319–324, 1993

Watson CPN, Babul N: Efficacy of oxycodone in neuropathic pain: a randomized trial in postherpetic neuralgia. Neurology 50:1833–1841, 1998

Watson CPN, Evans RJ: A comparative trial of amitriptyline and zimelidine in postherpetic neuralgia. Pain 23:387–394, 1985

Watson CPN, Evans RJ, Reed K, et al: Amitriptyline versus placebo in postherpetic neuralgia. Neurology 32:671–673, 1982

Watson CPN, Evans RJ, Watt VR: Postherpetic neuralgia and topical capsaicin. Pain 33:333–340, 1988

Watson CPN, Evans RJ, Watt VR: Amitriptyline versus maprotiline in postherpetic neuralgia, in Proceedings of the Ninth Annual Scientific Meeting of the American Pain Society. Skokie, IL, American Pain Society, 1990, pp 25–28

Weber RJ, Ikejiri B, Rice KC, et al: Opiate receptor mediated regulation of the immune response in vivo. NIDA Res Monogr 76:341–348, 1987

Willer JC, De Brouckner T, Bussel B, et al: Central analgesic effect of ketoprofen in humans—electrophysiological evidence for a supraspinal mechanism in a double-blind and cross-over study. Pain 38:1–7, 1989

Wolfe F, Cathey MA, Hawley DJ: A double-blind placebo controlled trial of fluoxetine in fibromyalgia. Scand J Rheumatol 23:255–259, 1994

Wolfe MN, Lichtenstein DR, Singh G: Gastroinstestinal toxicity of nonsteroidal anti-inflammatory drugs. N Engl J Med 340:1888–1899, 1999

World Health Organization: Cancer Pain Relief, 2nd Edition, With a Guide to Opioid Availability. Geneva, World Health Organization, 1996

Yaksh TL: An introductory perspective on the study of nociception and its modulation, in Anethesia: Biologic Foundations. Edited by Yaksh TL, Lynch C, Zapol W, et al. Philadelphia, PA, JB Lippincott, 1998, pp 471–483

Yang JC, Clark WC, Ngai SH, et al: Analgesic action and pharmacokinetics of morphine and diazepam in man: an evaluation by sensory decision theory. Anesthesiology 51:495–502, 1979

Yosselson-Superstine S, Lipman AG, Sanders SH: Adjunctive antianxiety agents in the management of chronic pain. Isr J Med Sci 21:113–117, 1985

Young RF, Rinaldi PC: Brain stimulation, in Neurosurgical Management of Pain. Edited by North RB, Levy RM. New York, Springer, 1997, pp 283–301

Zakrzewska JM, Chaudhry Z, Nurmikko TJ, et al: Lamotrigine (Lamictal) in refractory trigeminal neuralgia: results from a double-blind placebo-controlled crossover trial. Pain 73:223–230, 1997

Zenz M, Strumpf M, Tryba M: Long-term opioid therapy in patients with chronic nonmalignant pain. J Pain Symptom Manage 7:69–77, 1992

Ziegler DK: Opiate and opioid use in patients with refractory headache. Cephalalgia 14:5–10, 1994

Chapter 3

Psychogenic Models of Chronic Pain

A Selective Review and Critique

Randy S. Roth, Ph.D.

In this chapter, I selectively review the literature pertaining to the presumption of psychological causes for enigmatic chronic pain. For many pain scholars, the growth of psychogenic models of chronic pain has been born of necessity, by virtue of the belief that most chronic pain symptoms fit tenuously within a biomedical disease paradigm (Loeser 1991). The marriage of psychology and pain medicine recognizes the central role of psychological factors in understanding the persistence and morbidity associated with chronic pain (Gamsa 1994). Nonetheless, too often in the clinical setting, the etiology of pain is judged to be psychogenic, potential physiological parameters are devalued, and the patient and practitioner become embroiled in an adversarial relationship notable for disagreement, disdain, and distrust. Many of the negative outcomes for chronic pain treatment can be attributed to this failure of therapeutic rapport.

A biopsychosocial model of chronic pain has been proposed to broaden the perception of pain from a narrow sensorineural perspective to one that recognizes the mutually interactive contributions of biological, psychological, and environmental systems (Waddell 1996). Adopting a biopsychosocial perspective, I critically examine models of pain psychogenesis after reviewing the difficulties inherent in formulating a psychogenic pain diagnosis. I present data that challenge the conventional belief that numerous chronic pain patients have pain without a physiological substrate. I then consider three popular psychological models of psychogenic pain: the depiction of chronic pain 1) as a manifestation of psychological conversion (psychodynamic model), 2) as a symptom of depression (depression variant model), and 3) as the product of reinforcement mechanisms (operant model). As will be seen, the accumulating data suggest that as pure psychological causation of intractable pain becomes less defensible, the entanglement of psychological processes with pain physiology becomes more evident.

Prevalence of Psychogenic Pain

Published studies portray the uncertainty and diagnostic conundrums that are inherent when considering a differential diagnosis of psychogenic pain, somatoform pain disorder, and conversion pain disorder. Following a review of relevant studies, Dworkin and Caligor (1988) noted prevalence rates ranging from 16% to 53% for somatoform disorder among chronic pain populations. Both Katon et al. (1985) and Reich et al. (1983) reported that nearly one-third of their chronic pain samples merited a diagnosis of psychogenic pain disorder. However, Fishbain et al. (1986) found that fewer than 1% of their chronic pain patients met the criteria for psychogenic pain disorder, but nearly 40% had symptoms that suggested a conversion diagnosis. Atkinson et al. (1991) found no evidence of somatization among their population of chronic low back pain patients, but Owen-Salters et al. (1996) assessed 100% of their chronic back pain patients as having a somatoform pain disorder. These discrepant data parallel a marked disagreement among pain clinicians regarding the prevalence of psychogenic pain, with some observers noting rare occurrence (Gallagher 1999) and others arguing that most nonneurological pain is "hysterical" (Weintraub 1988).

Diagnosis of Psychogenic Pain

The inference of causality is at the heart of the dilemma for the clinician who must surmise a reasonable explanation for non-physiological pain. The elusive nature of pain and the ambiguities that commonly characterize the assessment of chronic pain frequently render the examiner with few objective (e.g., neurological, radiographic) benchmarks by which to determine a plausible medical diagnosis. The few pathognomonic clinical signs, in combination with knowledge deficits about mechanisms of pain, contribute to the elevation of subjective and cultural biases about chronic pain when considering causes of a patient's pain symptoms (Stratton-Hill 1995). The eventual diagnostic formulation will inevitably be influenced by the clinician's medical training and working paradigm for how to conceptualize intractable pain (Haddox 1996). As Calliet (1979) observed, each medical specialty comes to the enterprise of chronic pain with a certain idiosyncratic "tunnel vision" that governs the clinical interrogation, interpretation, and diagnosis of the pain patient.

Thus, diagnosing psychogenic pain can be as much in the eye of the beholder as it is a function of clinical findings and the patient's symptom presentation. It is easy, then, to understand why a psychodynamic psychiatrist, who attaches symbolic meaning to pain symptoms that are believed to represent unconscious emotional conflict, would be theoretically comfortable with diagnostic labels such as conversion disorder and somatoform disorder. However, a psychiatrist with a background in behavioral psychology, with its emphasis on pain as a behavior and the environmental stimuli that control it, would find these diagnostic categories clinically impractical and theoretically bankrupt.

The inherent subjectivity that frequently surrounds the psychiatric diagnosis of chronic pain is reflected in epidemiological and clinical studies and has raised concerns about the reliability of the standardized psychiatric taxonomy in this population (Fishbain et al. 1998a; King 1995). Changes in DSM-IV criteria (American Psychiatric Association 1994) reflect these clinical exigencies. DSM-III (American Psychiatric Association 1980) eliminated the diagnoses of conversion and hysteria when pain was the chief complaint but continued to endorse them in spirit with the designation *psychogenic pain disorder*. As Fishbain et al. (1998a) suggested, the diagnosis of psychogenic pain disorder required the clinician to infer the presence of an underlying psychological need or conflict and then ascertain whether it might bear causal relation to an overt pain report. Many pain clinicians found this determination excessively speculative and a poor fit for most of their patients. DSM-III-R (American Psychiatric Association 1987) changed *psychogenic* to *somatoform,* but the problems of clinical inference remained. Also, few pain researchers used the diagnostic option of somatoform pain disorder in their studies (King 1995). DSM-IV dropped the pejorative labels of *psychogenic* and *somatoform* and subsumed psychiatric pain diagnoses under the rubric *pain disorder,* which stratifies diagnostic options by three levels based on the presumed primacy of psychological factors contributing to pain. This taxonomy is more descriptive and broadens the effect of psychological factors to include the etiology, maintenance, severity, and/or exacerbation of pain symptoms (King 1995). This revised format appears to be more closely suited to the complexities and ambiguities of clinical pain, although whether it will fare any better than its predecessors remains to be seen.

Determining Psychological Causation

The domains of physiology and psychology are never more intertwined than during the clinical inquiry into chronic pain. A modern definition of pain now requires a consideration of affective, cognitive, and behavioral processes that interact with sensorineural pain transmission to produce human pain experience (Merskey and Bogduk 1994). Unlike other medical encounters, however, pain is an evanescent construct without physiological referent and always occurs within a psychological state as an experiential percept. Although diagnostic efforts often are successful in localizing tissue damage that may give rise to perceived pain, these assessment procedures frequently yield a correlation between pathophysiology and pain perception that is disappointingly low (Deyo 1996). Identifying nociception (i.e., pain transmission transduced from noxious stimuli) is the assumed target of clinical pain evaluation. Invariably, the credibility of the patient's pain complaint is contingent on a successful search.

Many chronic pain patients present with pain that evades a physiological determination or at least is difficult to reconcile in the face of normal neurological examination and negative radiography findings (Fordyce 1995). A clinical inference of psychogenesis generally is entertained in such cases, often to the dismay and frustration of the stigmatized patient and with potential catastrophic medicolegal and socioeconomic repercussions (Gallagher and Myers 1996). The high comorbidity of psychiatric disturbance among chronic pain patients and the fact that clinical pain is necessarily communicated by patient behavior may incline the clinician to consider emotional, personality, and behavioral factors when weighing causal parameters of pain perception.

Chronic pain comes to be construed as psychologically determined by multiple paths. First, the diagnosis of psychogenic pain is predicated on the exclusion of a physiological disturbance that has a credible relation to the patient's pain description. Establishing an association between tissue disturbance and patient self-report is customary for most medical examinations. However, in clinical pain, basic assumptions about a reliable interface between physiology and symptom complaint may prove misleading. For example, evidence of physiological abnormalities that presumably should provoke pain frequently do not. Striking evidence from radiological studies in the surgical literature attests to the nonlinear relation between tissue disturbance and pain perception. For example, 30%–40% of the records of asymptomatic patients who had computed tomography, myelography, and magnetic resonance imaging (MRI) indicated significant spinal abnormalities (Deyo 1996). Weinreb et al. (1989) reported that more than 50% of pregnant and asymptomatic women have abnormal disks on MRI. Spinal imaging of degenerative disk and joint diseases shows poor relation to clinical pain (Waddell 1991).

If the clinical investigation does not discern a plausible source of nociception, the obvious alternative is to view the patient's pain in terms of a disturbance in mood, personality, or motivation. This customary decision algorithm—rule out tissue pathology, thus rule in psychological etiology—is based on the entrenched Cartesian mind-body dualism that assumes a functional boundary between antecedent physiological events in the periphery and a separate interpretation of these events by an executive central processor: the mind. In this model, pain is contingent on peripheral activation. When a peripheral pain generator is absent, psychological mechanisms must be in operation. Although growing evidence from studies of pain perception challenge this anachronistic conceptualization of neurophysiology (Wall 1994), in the clinical setting, a dualistic paradigm continues to govern the study of chronic pain (Novy et al. 1995). The mere absence of detectable pathophysiology, however, is not sufficient foundation to establish a diagnosis of psychogenic pain, particularly without verification by independent psychological assessment.

Because the physician feels compelled to determine a definitive explanation for clinical pain when the etiology is not obvious, coupled with the presence of pain-related emotional distress and behavioral dysfunction, the role of psychogenesis may be overconsidered. In such circumstances, concurrent pain and severe psychological morbidity may suggest to the clinician that the psychological distress is causing the persistent pain. Although a determination of causality from the mere correlation of two variables is unjustified in statistical practice, it is understandable (although perhaps just as misleading) as a clinical inference within the demand characteristics of the clinical setting. The awareness that stress and coping strategies can alter pain intensity and disability (Jensen et al. 1991) only enhances the disposition to give causal weight to psychological factors when they coexist with chronic pain.

Physiological Sources of Psychogenic Pain

Neuroplasticity, Sensitization, and Pain Modulation

The presumption that many chronic pain patients have pain without physiological justification has been increasingly challenged. Wall (1994) exhorted pain clinicians to relinquish their adherence to a dualistic notion of pain and embrace a modern view of pain perception. This perspective derives from basic science investigations of pain neurophysiology that invoke the principles of neuroplasticity, sensitization, and pain modulation to identify mechanisms of pain perception independent of tissue damage (Coderre et al. 1993; Fields and Basbaum 1994). Peripheral and central mechanisms devoted to pain perception are now known to be dynamic and mutually interactive. Most notably, in response to persistent nociceptive input (particularly when the integrity of the nervous system is compromised), the nervous system biases toward enhanced nociception and pain experience by prompting functional and morphological changes in neural structures and pathways. Prolonged acute pain with associated nociception can promote changes in both the peripheral and the central nervous systems, producing heightened pain perception via reduced threshold activation for pain-mediating nerve cells (e.g., sensitization) to both noxious and innocuous stimuli. Sensitization of peripheral afferents can be shown following tissue damage or nerve injury and may be sustained by peptides and transmitter agents that result from inflammation and tissue damage or release from the afferent's own terminals. The hyperalgesia (i.e., exaggerated pain response) typically observed after injury is believed to result from sensitization.

Sensitization also occurs at the level of the spinal cord. Constant but fixed nociceptive input received by first-order central cells located in the dorsal horn promotes increased and enhanced firing of these cells or "windup" (Coderre et al. 1993). In this way, pain may become "centralized" whereby spinal pain transmission neurons acquire a lowered activation threshold and thus are triggered by large-diameter afferents carrying mechanical (e.g., movement, innocuous touch) rather than pain information. Also, evidence from classical conditioning studies indicates that these first-order central cells can learn to fire in response to environmental stimuli that were previously associated with nociception and in the absence of peripheral afferent provocation (Duncan et al. 1987). Even more astonishing are recent data from the study of phantom limb pain (Flor et al. 1995b). Patients with phantom pain, but not those with phantom phenomena, had cortical reorganization of the primary somatosensory cortex, suggesting that central plasticity also may extend to the brain after persistent pain. The authors speculated that some aspects of phantom pain might actually result from these cortical changes.

Neuroplastic changes that result in an enhanced pain experience serve the critical signaling function of informing the organism of potential or actual threat to biological integrity. But an animal in pain is at risk, so it is not surprising that the neuropathways relevant to pain transmission are susceptible to modulation

(Fields and Basbaum 1994). The possibility of a central locus for pain modulation was first suggested by the gate control theory of pain (Melzack and Wall 1965). This theory has proven extraordinarily robust in providing a blueprint for the neuropsychological mechanisms of pain perception. The authors hypothesized peripheral and central mechanisms of pain modulation subserved by a complex interplay of neural circuitry that facilitates both peripheral and descending inhibition and that acts to either excite or inhibit relevant spinal neurons that are responsible for pain transmission.

Pain modulation can be mounted by neural activity in several ways. Stimulation of large mechanoreceptors, specialized for innocuous sensation, appears to inhibit the activation of spinal pain transmission neurons that are concurrently receiving nociceptive input. This has been suggested as the mechanism by which massage, cold packs, transcutaneous nerve stimulation, and spinal cord stimulation reduce pain. Separate ascending spinothalamic pathways appear to carry different aspects of pain (Fields and Basbaum 1994). A lateral tract relays pain information to the thalamus and conveys the sensory-discriminative aspect of pain. A second, more medial tract, which collateralizes to various brain structures in the midbrain, medulla, and limbic system, is thought to convey the affective-motivational aspect of pain. Of note, this latter pathway innervates brain centers, such as the hypothalamus, that have been implicated in the regulation of mood, attention, and cognition. The anxiety, fear, and motive to avoid that are associated with pain may reside in this spinothalamic connection.

More profound pain modulation appears to rest in the activation of specific brain centers that produce analgesia when electrically or chemically stimulated. Reynolds (1969) was the first to report that the brain can be the origin of analgesia for peripheral pain. Numerous laboratories have replicated this breakthrough discovery and expanded the brain mapping to identify those structures and their descending pathways that facilitate central pain suppression (Fields and Basbaum 1994). To this end, current evidence indicates that the midbrain periaqueductal gray, the rostral medulla in the midline nucleus raphe magnus, and the dorsolateral pontine tegmentum all have the capability to exert inhibitory control on peripheral nociception. This supraspinal inhibition is conveyed via descending pathways whose end terminals synapse with spinal neurons and peripheral afferents in the dorsal horn. These descending pathways are mediated, at least in part, by the biogenic amines serotonin and norepinephrine (Basbaum et al. 1983). These data have suggested a central role for neurotransmitter systems that have been implicated in the biology of psychiatric disorders but now seem integral to pain modulatory mechanisms as well. Conversely, evidence suggests that endogenous opioids, known to be important in mediating neural mechanisms of pain modulation (Watkins and Mayer 1982), may have an equally critical role in the regulation of psychiatric disorders (Cohen et al. 1984).

The unveiling of a pain modulatory apparatus within the nervous system, and the evidence that the nervous system is mutable when bombarded by ongoing nociception, has important lessons for clinical pain. First, it is clear that ongoing acute pain increases the potential for chronic pain, resulting in the central excitation of pain that does not require a persistent peripheral pain generator. A recent clinical application of these data has been the use of preemptive analgesia to reduce postoperative pain (Niv and Devor 1996). Neuroplasticity also serves as the backdrop for the investigation of central nervous system dysregulation as the etiology of intractable pain syndromes heretofore considered purely psychiatric, such as fibromyalgia and reflex sympathetic dystrophy (Crofford et al. 1994; Gracely et al. 1992). Second, psychological processes governed by brain centers integral to stress and mood functioning are "hard-wired" within pain pathways that inform higher neurological structures of the presence of pain. These structures are responsible for the unpleasantness and aversion that accompanies noxious stimulation. Thus, the Cartesian split between psyche and soma, on which clinical decision making for pain has relied, is not only therapeutically misdirected but also anatomically nonsensical.

Musculoskeletal Pain

Musculoskeletal pain disorders (e.g., myofascial pain) are a second and common source of enigmatic chronic pain (Bonica and

Sola 1992). Musculoskeletal disorders are a major cause of health care use and functional disability (Badley et al. 1994). Among patients with chronic pain, 90% localize their pain to the musculoskeletal system rather than the nervous system (Andersson et al. 1993). This finding is consistent with data from the surgical literature that find a very low prevalence of disk herniation and spinal pathology for patients with low back pain (Deyo 1996). However, despite the prevalence of musculoskeletal pain, and long-standing pleas for its recognition as a valid and treatable origin of chronic pain (Bonica 1957), a veritable schism divides the thinking of pain scholars on the nature and legitimacy of chronic soft-tissue pain. This controversy reveals much about the role of paradigmatic thinking for an understanding of the variability in clinical inference observed across pain practitioners (Haddox 1996).

A vocal and prolific group of investigators, arguing from a traditional neurological-surgical perspective, have cast doubt on the medical validity of pathophysiological determinants of chronic musculoskeletal pain, for example, in the case of chronic low back pain (Waddell 1996). These investigators believe that medically defensible origins of nociception for chronic low back pain are limited to serious spinal lesions (e.g., spinal stenosis, spondylolisthesis, vertebral fracture and disease) and nerve root disturbance (e.g., herniated disk). Pain and corollary symptoms that are outside the confines of neurological impairment (e.g., nondermatomal sensory loss) are construed as *nonorganic* (Waddell et al. 1989). The remaining chronic low back pain patients, which includes the vast majority of these patients, are said to have *nonspecific* low back pain (Fordyce 1995), defined as a "simple backache" that is commonplace, self-limiting, and benign (Waddell 1996).

With the epidemic rise in back pain disability among Western industrialized nations, and given the belief that nonspecific low back pain has no organic basis, these investigators have turned to environmental (e.g., compensation) and psychological factors to explain the prevalence of disabling back pain. This perspective was recently formalized in a monograph on back pain in the workplace (Fordyce 1995). The panel recommended that patients with industrial back pain that persists beyond 6 weeks are to be considered "activity intolerant," are to be denied further medical attention for their pain (because they have a social problem, not a medical illness), and are to be reclassified as unemployed rather than disabled. Although seemingly harsh, these recommendations avoid the more pejorative view of pain researchers who consider nonspecific low back pain to reflect "hysteria" (Weintraub 1988), malingering (Awerbuch 1992), or abnormal illness behavior (Pilowsky 1978).

An alternative view of nonneurological low back pain emphasizes the musculoskeletal dysfunction associated with myofascial trigger points (Simons et al. 1999). Rosomoff et al. (1989) carefully examined patients with chronic neck and low back pain who were referred for pain rehabilitation for "chronic intractable benign pain." The authors found that 97% of these patients had evidence of trigger points or tender points, most had reduced range of motion, and nearly 50% complained of nondermatomal sensory loss. The authors concluded that many patients with nonspecific spinal pain actually have myofascial pain.

In a similar report, Hendler and Kozikowski (1993) found that 66% of referred chronic pain patients had been underdiagnosed for organic disease, and myofascial pain was the most common of the missed diagnoses. Despite these studies, several investigators continue to dispute the medical viability of trigger points as a source of pain, pointing to the absence of a model of pathophysiology for myofascial pain (Weintraub 1988). However, data from animal models and clinical studies are beginning to clarify the electrophysiological and biochemical aberrations associated with myofascial trigger points and the mechanisms underlying referred pain (Mense 1994; Simons et al. 1999).

The question of chronicity has been a serious impediment to a wider acceptance of myofascial pain as the etiology for chronic back pain. As is well known, soft-tissue injuries usually are self-limiting, but muscle pain can be persistent. Nearly 30% of the patients with a first onset of back pain continue to complain of significant pain at 1 year (Cherkin et al. 1996). At the neurophysiological level, Mense (1994) used an animal model of persistent muscle pain (e.g., experimental myositis) and described changes in spinal neuron excitability after sustained afferent nociception from muscle resulting in central sensitization. In a clinical application of this model, Bendtsen et al. (1996) found evidence for altered nociceptive processing with reduced pain tolerance in a sample of chronic myofascial pain patients. The authors speculated that sensitized dorsal horn neurons might be responsible for the chronicity of myofascial pain.

Clinically, Simons et al. (1999) emphasized the role of perpetuating factors, such as skeletal asymmetry, nutritional deficiencies, muscle overuse, and emotional stress, in the maintenance of myofascial pain following its onset. Altered musculoskeletal biomechanics also can contribute to the maintenance of myofascial pain (Calliet 1979). In this regard, Greenman (1996) described common somatic dysfunctions (e.g., skeletal malalignment, joint restrictions) that sustain musculoskeletal restrictions and complicate the treatment of myofascial pain. Janda (1994) highlighted the muscle inhibition and imbalances that accrue from soft-tissue injury, with resultant derangement of musculoskeletal regulation, that also serve as perpetuating factors in chronic soft-tissue pain. All of these dynamic functional changes, which often arise over time after an injury to the musculoskeletal system, encourage self-perpetuating cycles of pain and dysfunction.

Myofascial pain syndromes often are diagnosed as psychological pain (Shapiro and Teasell 1998). The poorly localized, diffuse, and nondermatomal radiation of referred pain that characterizes nociception from muscles can be easily misinterpreted as nonanatomical (Mense 1994). In addition, the diagnosis of myofascial pain, with its pattern of radiating or referred pain from trigger points, is extremely confusing for the clinician not acquainted with the numerous myofascial syndromes. As a result, myofascial pain from specific muscles can be readily mistaken for alternative pain syndromes. Common examples include the piriformis for a radiculopathy (Durrani and Winnie 1991), the sternocleidomastoid for atypical facial pain (Travell 1981), the splenius capitis/cervicis for occipital neuralgia (Graff-Radford et al. 1986), and the upper trapezius for a migraine headache (Simons et al. 1999). Failure to respond to interventions (e.g., surgery) for the diagnosed disorder, when the patient actually has myofascial pain, can lead to suspicions about the patient's motivation. More often, the patient is simply left without a clear diagnosis.

The issue of specificity of diagnosis can have far-reaching clinical implications when considering myofascial pain. Faucett (1994) observed that myofascial pain patients, when compared with arthritis patients, reported significantly more conflict about their pain with significant others, perceived less social network support, and were more depressed. The author suggested that the lack of objective physical findings in myofascial pain might have led relatives and friends to question the validity of the patient's pain.

Roth et al. (1998) compared a group of myofascial pain patients with a group of chronic pain patients with diagnosed "objective" pain syndromes (e.g., radiculopathy, rheumatoid arthritis) regarding their understanding of and beliefs about their pain. Myofascial pain patients were less accurate in identifying their diagnosis, more likely to think that their pain was more serious than physicians had suggested, and significantly more dissatisfied with the lack of information provided by their physicians. In a follow-up study, Geisser and Roth (1998) stratified chronic pain patients into "agree," "disagree," and "uncertain" groups based on their knowledge of and agreement with their pain diagnosis. Myofascial pain patients again were more likely to disagree with their pain diagnosis and reported the highest levels of pain intensity and affective distress compared with chronic pain patients who were accurate or simply uncertain of their diagnosis. In addition, patients who were uncertain of or disagreed with their diagnosis were more likely to believe that their pain represented a signal of harm or physiological damage. Both groups also favored the use of maladaptive pain coping strategies. A hierarchical regression analysis found that pain disability was best predicted by the belief about pain as a signal of harm, with the lack of knowledge regarding diagnosis, affective distress, and catastrophic worry about pain also contributing significantly to the variance in disability. Pain intensity had no relation to disability. The authors concluded that uncertainty about one's pain diagnosis might dispose a patient to dysfunctional pain beliefs and maladaptive pain coping strategies that foster disability.

Psychological Models of Chronic Pain

Psychodynamic Model

The psychoanalytic theory of psychogenic pain begins with Freud (1937), who appealed to the mechanism of conversion to explain pain symptoms among his patients with hysteria. Under such circumstances, the model asserts that unconscious, ego-dystonic, and anxiety-riddled conflicts and needs are transformed into bodily pain as a means to restore psychic homeostasis. The symbolic theme of the precipitating unconscious motive is preserved in the form the pain adopts (e.g., sexual abuse manifesting as pelvic pain). In an important elaboration of this model, Engel (1959) provided an in-depth description of the developmental antecedents and adult character structure associated with the "pain-prone personality." Although the model's empirical validity is in question (Turk and Flor 1984), Freud is rightfully credited with drawing attention to the central contribution of psychological processes to somatic medicine. The psychoanalytic notion of persistent pain as an expression of psychological disturbance is deeply embedded in the cultural zeitgeist and attests to Freud's enduring legacy. Of critical importance, his conversion thesis armed clinical medicine with a shorthand diagnostic fallback in cases in which somatic symptoms defy medical scrutiny.

Consistent with psychoanalytic ideology, psychogenic pain is understood to result from developmental experiences that enhance the prominence of pain in childhood and give rise to the role of pain as a servant to adult defenses. Engel (1959) proposed that adverse events in childhood engender, for the child, strong and aberrant associations between pain and affect. For example, when child-parent interactions disproportionately surround themes of punishment and abuse, the child begins to associate punishment (pain) with bonding with the love object (pleasure). As adults, these individuals are said to seek masochistic relationships that reenact these childhood transactions. Furthermore, pain in childhood is linked to "badness" and guilt during punishment, the parental display of aggression and power, and the real or imagined loss of a love object. These developmental pain-affect connections lay the foundation for adult coping and the invocation of pain under conditions of psychological strain. A "pain-prone" adult who has unbearable guilt, the urge to aggress, or suffers interpersonal loss will be inclined to resurrect somatic pain as a savior from intolerable psychic distress. Thus, psychogenic pain can serve as a defense mechanism through its function as a diversion from unbearable affect, in the expiation of unrelenting guilt, or to obtain gratification in response to underlying dependency needs.

Because the actual mechanism of conversion is impossible to examine directly, psychodynamic writers have attempted to verify their model empirically by examining the premorbid history and personality traits of patients who have pain without organic findings. Unfortunately, the large majority of these studies involved single or extended case reports (Tinling and Klein 1966) or uncontrolled clinical investigations (Violon 1985) that provide sparse experimental data. General reviews of the psychodynamic model of chronic pain (Gamsa 1994; Turk and Flor 1984) and a more specific reevaluation of Engel's thesis (Roy 1985) have all concluded that no consistent empirical evidence supports the model's applicability to most chronic pain patients. For example, studies exploring a linear relationship between a history of parental punishment or childhood deprivation and chronic pain have obtained mixed results. In one of the few controlled comparisons, Adler et al. (1989) found a high prevalence of parental and emotional abuse in patients with "psychogenic" pain compared with a group of patients with organic pain, other psychosomatic symptoms, or medical disorders. These results must be viewed cautiously, however, because the measurement methodology was not standardized and the sample size was small. Conversely, Gamsa (1990; Gamsa and Vikis-Freibergs 1991) and Merskey et al. (1987) found no evidence of an association between abnormal childhood development and various pain parameters for chronic pain patients when compared with control subjects.

In a similar vein, anecdotal accounts from psychoanalytic reports have attributed a causal role to personality traits such as narcissism (Blazer 1980–81), aggressiveness (Tinling and Klein 1966), the inability to express intense affect (Beutler et al. 1986), and overcompensated dependency needs (Van Houdenhove

1986) when analyzing clinical cases of unexplained intractable pain. However, a controlled study that specifically assessed traits such as emotional repression, perceived independence, and the expression of affect found no relation between these variables and chronic pain (Gamsa and Vikis-Freibergs 1991). Cox et al. (1978) compared the personality profiles of patients with chronic pain of known organicity with those of patients with chronic pain without a clear organic basis and found no differences between the groups. Wade et al. (1992) found that the large majority of chronic pain patients show normal personality functioning on standardized psychological tests. Tauschke et al. (1990) compared chronic pain patients and psychiatric patients and found that the former group had less evidence of abnormal childhood rearing and used more mature defense mechanisms.

A central tenet of the psychodynamic model of psychogenesis for pain draws a symbolic relation between the body site of pain and the nature of the unconscious conflict or developmental trauma that gives rise to it. The relationship between childhood sexual abuse and chronic pelvic pain in women is perhaps the most obvious example of this extension of the conversion hypothesis (E. A. Walker et al. 1988). Early reports from the gynecology literature noted a particularly high prevalence of childhood sexual abuse among women with chronic pelvic pain, particularly in those alleged to have pelvic pain without an apparent medical cause (Reiter et al. 1991). These studies are difficult to interpret in support of a specific etiological role for childhood sexual abuse in the development of chronic pelvic pain because of the significant base rate of childhood sexual abuse in the general population (Briere and Runtz 1991). Moreover, data suggest that the long-held assumption that most chronic pelvic pain is "enigmatic" (Ranaer et al. 1980) may need reexamination. Beard et al. (1984) reported that 84% of women with a history of chronic pelvic pain without obvious pathology had clinical findings of large dilated pelvic veins and vascular stasis, suggesting that pelvic congestion may have been a cause of their pain. More recently, Punch et al. (1994) noted that 21% of 160 consecutive women with chronic pelvic pain were found to have myofascial pain as their primary pain diagnosis. Of those patients for whom follow-up data were available,

70% experienced significant or total pain relief following physical therapy. Taken together, these findings suggest that many women with a diagnosis of psychogenic pelvic pain may actually have treatable medical disorders that account for their pain symptoms.

More pertinent to the presumption of childhood sexual abuse as a direct cause of chronic pelvic pain is the degree to which childhood sexual abuse serves as proxy for other trauma and family variables that actually account for adult morbidity (Rind et al. 1998). In this regard, Engels et al. (1994) showed that women who report a history of childhood sexual abuse or physical abuse also are more likely to have witnessed family violence, have alcoholic parents, and come from divorced homes. These authors also found that physical abuse was the strongest predictor of adult psychiatric disorders. In a comprehensive meta-analytic review, Rind et al. (1998) concluded that the observed relationship between childhood sexual abuse and adult psychological maladjustment becomes nonsignificant when relevant family environmental factors are controlled. Several multivariate studies of chronic pelvic pain also have found that childhood physical abuse but not sexual abuse is significantly associated with pain, affective distress, and disability among this population (Rapkin et al. 1990; E. A. Walker et al. 1997). These results raise questions about a significant correlation between childhood sexual abuse and chronic pelvic pain and, by implication, the symbolism hypothesis of psychogenic pain expression.

As can be seen, the psychodynamic model of psychogenic pain has had seminal historical significance and has received widespread acceptance within the culture and clinical medicine. Its effect on pain medicine has been equally profound. The notion of psychological pain in its modern version would be unthinkable apart from psychoanalytic theory. But the contribution of the psychodynamic model has been double-edged, because it automatically presumes psychogenesis in cases in which pain does not ascribe to the classic (and outdated) view of pain mechanisms. The emphasis on inference and the speculative nature of the psychodynamic inquiry raise serious concerns of construct validity when considering a cause of psychogenic pain (Gallagher 1999). More important, the psychodynamic model of pain has failed to withstand the test of empirical scrutiny. In addition, with the ascendance of behavioral and cognitive-behavioral theories of human behavior, the popularity of psychoanalytic thinking within mainstream psychology has been declining. Thus, it is not surprising that published pain studies that consider a psychoanalytic perspective have steadily declined in the past 15 years (Gamsa 1994).

Depression Variant Model

Symptoms of depression are the most predictable psychological disturbance associated with chronic pain (Atkinson et al. 1991; Romano and Turner 1985). As pain persists beyond the acute stage, depressive symptoms proliferate in most pain patients. Rates of depression are higher among chronic pain patients than in other medically ill patients (Banks and Kerns 1996). The prevalence of depressive symptoms among chronic pain patients varies across studies from 10% to 100% (Romano and Turner 1985), with more reasonable estimates suggesting 30%–54% (Banks and Kerns 1996). The variability in rates of depression across these studies likely reflects differences in patient selection, clinical setting, measurement methodology, and the diagnostic rigor by which depression is defined (e.g., symptoms vs. disorder) (Crook et al. 1986; Romano and Turner 1985). Recent evidence indicates that approximately one-third of chronic pain patients have major depressive disorder (Geisser et al. 1997).

Depression has been consistently found to increase morbidity in patients with chronic pain. Compared with a nondepressed cohort, chronic pain patients with depression report more severe pain, report a higher frequency of pain behavior, and show greater physical, vocational, and psychosocial disability (Dworkin et al. 1986; Haythornthwaite et al. 1991; Keefe et al. 1986). They are also more likely to either drop out of treatment or respond poorly to intervention (Blanchard et al. 1982; Kerns and Haythornthwaite 1988).

Based on the considerable probability of comorbid depression in chronic pain patients who present without a verifiable level of organicity, several authors have proposed a model that views chronic pain as a variant of depression (Blumer and Heilbronn

1982). In this model, chronic pain is conceptualized as an affective spectrum disorder in which pain is viewed, with depressive symptoms, as a synchronous expression of an underlying or "muted" depression. Several lines of evidence support the model. Family members of chronic pain patients have a high prevalence of affective disorder (Blumer and Heilbronn 1982). In addition, Blumer et al. (1982) found that chronic pain patients have a positive response to biological markers for depression (e.g., dexamethasone suppression). Blumer and Heilbronn (1982) also noted the growing empirical support for the efficacy of antidepressant therapy in controlling chronic pain (Max et al. 1987) as evidence for the mutual nature of chronic pain and depression. These data collectively bolstered the view that chronic pain without verifiable pathophysiology is best construed as a variant of depression.

Perhaps the strongest data to support the notion that depression causes pain in most chronic pain patients derive from studies that examined pain complaints among populations of depressed patients. In an early study, Ward et al. (1979) recruited community members with depression and anxiety. Of 16 individuals who were screened for severe depression, all admitted to problems with persistent pain over the previous 6 months. Treatment with the tricyclic antidepressant (TCA) doxepin significantly reduced in linear fashion both depression and pain. Von Knorring et al. (1983) observed that 57% of depressed psychiatric inpatients reported problems with pain. In an epidemiological study, Wells et al. (1989) reported that 35% of the patients with depressive symptoms complained of somatic pain. In a prospective study, Magni et al. (1994) found that a diagnosis of depression significantly predicted the occurrence of chronic pain 8 years later. In a study with remarkably similar results, Atkinson et al. (1991) noted that in men with chronic low back pain, assessed for lifetime and prior 6-month prevalence of psychiatric disturbance, 40% had a history of a depressive episode. The mean for the first episode of depression was nearly 8 years before the first onset of pain.

Blumer and Heilbronn (1982) presented the most complete argument for the view of chronic pain as depression. These authors acknowledged their indebtedness to Engel (1959) and his description of the "pain-prone personality," whereby causal significance was attributed to developmental trauma and adult personality traits to explain psychogenic pain. Blumer and Heilbronn modernized Engel's thesis by incorporating available evidence from neurophysiological studies of pain mechanisms. These studies had strongly implicated a critical role for biogenic amines (e.g., serotonin, norepinephrine) in mediating endogenous pain modulation. These neurotransmitters were already known to play a central role in the regulation of affect. In reconceptualizing chronic pain as a "pain-prone disorder," the authors hypothesized that a biological vulnerability to depression and personality characteristics that derive from psychodynamic conceptualizations of depression (e.g., guilt) converge in the chronic pain patient.

Blumer's research was both provocative and pivotal as it generated a serious and productive debate on the relation between chronic pain and depression. However, although it may correctly describe a subset of chronic pain patients, the pain-as-depression model appears to be overly restrictive as a general model of chronic pain (Novy et al. 1995). That chronic pain cannot be summarily reduced to depression is attested by the fact that many chronic pain patients are not depressed. Moreover, Romano and Turner (1985) correctly noted that the presence of vegetative signs of depression among chronic pain patients does not distinguish them from other psychiatric or medical patients and thus is of questionable diagnostic significance. Turk and Salovey (1984) cogently reexamined the empirical grounds on which Blumer's original studies were based, noting methodological shortcomings in study design, inappropriate statistical analyses, and a lack of parsimony in drawing clinical inferences from the data. Furthermore, subsequent empirical studies failed to replicate the evidence for biological markers that characterize chronic pain as depression (France et al. 1984).

The empirical verification of Blumer's model is important. When pain is misattributed to depression, patients may become frustrated and defensive or feel betrayed by and alienated from the health care system, adding to increased affective distress (Reid et al. 1991). To this end, the preponderance of available data confirms that most chronic pain patients experience depression consequent to the onset of pain, with some episodes occurring as many as 5 years later (Atkinson et al. 1991; Fishbain et al. 1997). Longitudinal studies of patients with rheumatoid arthritis, who were asked to monitor pain and mood on a daily basis, found that degree of depression most frequently followed rather than preceded increased pain (Affleck et al. 1992). In contrast to previously cited studies (e.g., Magni et al. 1994), several studies have failed to support the contention that depression is a risk factor for the onset of pain (Atkinson et al. 1991; Von Korff et al. 1993). In addition, successful treatment of pain leads to resolution of depression in a high percentage of chronic pain patients, even when the treatment does not include antidepressant therapy (Maruta et al. 1989).

If we assume the converse of Blumer's model—that pain is most often primary to depression—then we would expect a significant association between indices of pain severity and greater depressive disorder. Indeed, duration of pain, severity of perceived pain, extent of bodily pain, and number of pain conditions are all associated with either a higher risk for depression or greater severity of depressive disorder (Fishbain et al. 1997). Additional studies point to sociodemographic variables as potential mediators of the correlation between depression and chronic pain. Among chronic pain patients, depression has been linked to young age (Haythornthwaite et al. 1991), low educational achievement, single marital status, unemployment (Averill et al. 1996), female gender, rural residence (Magni et al. 1994), and low social support (Kerns and Haythornthwaite 1988).

Any discussion of chronic pain and depression must include an examination of the effectiveness of antidepressants in treating chronic pain. Early investigations, many of which were uncontrolled clinical trials, that demonstrated the analgesic efficacy of antidepressants for chronic pain frequently emphasized the association between reduced pain and improved depressive symptoms (Feinmann 1985). These studies surmised that a decrease in depression likely mediates the analgesic effect of antidepressants. The inference that depression mediates analgesia when pain is effectively treated by antidepressants was illustrated in a report by Turkington (1980). After the pain and mood disturbance in a group of diabetic patients with painful neuropathy and concurrent depression were treated successfully with antidepressants, the author concluded that, for these patients, "depression (was) masquerading as diabetic neuropathy" (p. 1147).

Incontrovertible evidence from animal models and human clinical studies now indicates that antidepressants have analgesic properties apart from their antidepressant effect (Max 1995; Onghena and Van Houdenhove 1992). In an important study noteworthy for its experimental design, Max et al. (1987) recruited 29 patients with severe diabetic neuropathy, confirmed by electromyography, for a double-blind, crossover, placebo-controlled trial to assess the analgesic benefits of the TCA amitriptyline (average dose, 90 mg). Each patient was carefully screened for psychological impairment. Approximately half of the patients were found to be clinically depressed. Amitriptyline was significantly effective in reducing pain compared with placebo. More importantly, the rate of pain reduction with amitriptyline was equivalent for both the depressed and the nondepressed subjects, indicating that changes in a preexisting mood condition were not necessary to explain pain reduction.

Several reviews have summarized the expanding literature on antidepressant treatment of chronic pain (Jung et al. 1997; Max 1995; Onghena and Van Houdenhove 1992). Some general findings emerge from this literature. Antidepressants produce pain relief in patients without depressed mood and, interestingly, are equally effective in patients with psychogenic and physiologically based chronic pain (Fishbain et al. 1998b). Clinically, "mixed" TCAs (e.g., nortriptyline) appear to be superior to more selective agents (e.g., fluoxetine), but all categories have shown analgesic properties. In contrast to the typical action of antidepressants for the treatment of affective disorder, analgesic response occurs within days rather than weeks and at a dosage considerably lower than that recommended for depression. Antidepressants have been clinically effective in a wide range of pain syndromes, including headache, diabetic neuropathy, postherpetic neuralgia, central pain syndromes, fibromyalgia, chronic pelvic pain, and low back pain with sciatica (Atkinson et al. 1998; Max 1995; E. A. Walker et al. 1993). In the laboratory, TCAs are known to potentiate opioid analgesia in animals (Levine et al. 1986). At this time, the exact mechanisms by which antidepressants effect pain reduction are not known. Possible mediating mechanisms include the inhibition of spinal pain transmission neurons through descending pathways or local action, activation of endogenous opioids, blockade of sodium channels, or reduction in efferent sympathetic outflow (Max 1995).

Data from laboratory studies of pain tolerance among depressed patients suggest that the interaction of pain and depression is more complicated than it appears. Given the considerable effect of depression on pain morbidity, it is not surprising that induction of a depressed mood among healthy volunteers results in an increase in somatic focus and complaints of discomfort (Salovey and Birnbaum 1989). However, paradoxical findings from several laboratories have been reported in which depressed patients have a heightened threshold for experimentally induced pain compared with nondepressed control subjects (Lautenbacher et al. 1994). Importantly, these subjects do not show corollary change in general sensory responsiveness. How these data reconcile with findings from clinical studies is unclear but does point to the complexity of the pain-depression connection.

In summary, a model that reduces the experience of chronic pain to a variant of depression clearly is not supported by available research. It is similarly obvious that depression is a significant comorbid problem for many chronic pain patients. Individuals with a history of affective disorder are vulnerable to the experience of pain symptoms, and the presence of depression in a chronic pain patient can significantly complicate clinical morbidity and pain treatment outcome. Clinically, depression appears to amplify the perception of pain. As a result, successful treatment of chronic pain often requires particular attention to depression as a target of intervention (Sullivan et al. 1992). Indeed, different variables may be associated with positive outcome for depressed compared with nondepressed chronic pain patients (Dworkin et al. 1986).

Operant Model

The seminal writings of Fordyce (1976) introduced the principles of learning theory to the conceptualizations of chronic pain. Borrowing from the operant conditioning studies of Skinner (1953), Fordyce correctly observed that, as pain is always communicated via behavior, the occurrence and frequency of "pain behaviors" are susceptible to the influence of environmental stimuli. Noting that chronic pain persists beyond the typical course of an acute injury, and invoking the conventional wisdom that most chronic pain exists in a vacuum of pathophysiology, Fordyce proposed that the functional control of pain behavior transfers from antecedent nociception, which results from an inciting injury, to reinforcing consequences mediated by the social environment (Fordyce 1979). Thus, the persistence of pain disability is attributed to the consequences of pain expression, such as the receipt of financial reward or comforting spousal attention or the avoidance of aversive conditions such as a stressful work setting or unpleasant interpersonal obligations, through the operation of positive and negative reinforcement, respectively.

The clinical implication of the operant perspective is a focus on contingency management, or altering the relation between pain behavior and its environmental effects (Latimer 1982). Pain medications that are commonly administered as needed are dispensed on a time-contingent basis, reasoning that the reduction in pain that follows analgesic consumption can serve as a negative reinforcer for (and increase the frequency of) the pain behavior that precedes it. Similarly, exercise regimens are restructured so that the patient is expected to exercise to a quota rather than to pain tolerance, based on the hypothesis that the patient who terminates activity when pain increases, and thus avoids the aversive stimulus of pain, is being negatively reinforced for "activity intolerance" (Fordyce 1995). Pain program staff and spouses of pain patients are educated to differentially attend to health behaviors (e.g., increased activity) and ignore expressions of pain. A clinical demonstration of the efficacy of this treatment model, inspired by operant theory, was first reported by Fordyce et al. (1973), who noted increased activity and decreased pain in 36 inpatients undergoing chronic pain rehabilitation. These findings were followed by a proliferation of pain programs and published studies that heralded the effectiveness of "behavior therapy" for the treatment of "operant pain" (Latimer 1982; Turner and Chapman 1982;

Ziesat et al. 1979). Suggesting that the operant model had stimulated a fundamental paradigm shift for the study of chronic pain is not an overstatement.

The operant model of chronic pain found a welcome reception among pain researchers and clinicians, occurring in step with the growing application of behavior therapy to medical disorders in the 1970s. The model also was consistent with the concepts of "sick role" (Mechanic 1962) and "illness behavior" (Pilowsky 1978) that drew attention to chronically ill patients who had severe dysfunction, frequent health care use, and noticeable discrepancies between symptom presentation and medical findings. Early case reports (Fordyce et al. 1982), single group outcome studies (Anderson et al. 1977), and a few controlled investigations (Linton and G'otestam 1985) provided encouraging support for the operant perspective. Insidiously, for many clinicians the orientation to the chronic pain patient was transformed. Interest in pain behavior replaced a central concern with pain experience. In some instances, patients receiving pain-related compensation or with pending litigation, being deemed untreatable, were excluded from pain rehabilitation (Roberts and Reinhardt 1980). For many patients, the exclusive attention to their behavior rather than their pain experience was confusing and disconcerting.

Unfortunately, critical reviews of behavioral pain treatment programs have concluded that even though positive outcomes can be achieved, serious methodological problems raise questions about the basic assumptions on which operant programs are based (Latimer 1982; Schmidt 1987). Chief among these concerns is that these purported "behavioral" programs actually comprised multidisciplinary interventions whereby patients received a wide variety of therapies (e.g., physical therapy, occupational therapy, individual and group therapy, vocational counseling) (Turner and Chapman 1982). The attribution of treatment gains to the operant component of the program was speculative and misleading (Linton and G'otestam 1985; Schmidt 1987). Studies that have attempted a component analysis of multidisciplinary pain treatment did not support a particular advantage of operant therapy for reducing pain disability when compared with other pain modalities (Heinrich et al. 1985; Turner et al. 1990). Still other studies have reported negative results for the operant treatment of pain (Schmidt et al. 1989).

The operant pain behavior construct has become the target of heated debate and reexamination on both theoretical and empirical grounds (Turk and Flor 1987). As Lacey (1985) observed, a critical conceptual problem with the operant model of pain pertains to its apparent confusion of topography and function in defining an operant. Skinner (1935) defined operant behavior on the basis of its functional relationship to the environment. Borrowing from the classic operant experimental paradigm, a rat can press a bar in many ways (topography), but each form of behavior shares a common effect on the environment (activation of the food dispenser) that defines the bar press as an operant. In other words, operants are a class of topographical behaviors that share in common a singular and easily defined effect on the environment. The operant pain model has argued from a converse vantage—the defining property is the behavior (e.g., pain behavior) rather than how the behavior brings about a common environmental consequence. This is illustrated by the dogmatic assertion that "pain behaviors are operants" (Fordyce 1979, p. 661). For example, consider the difficulty in interpreting a common environmental consequence when pain behaviors for one patient result in spouse solicitousness and for another precipitate spouse withdrawal (Lacey 1985).

A second conceptual problem with the operant pain model concerns the application of the principle of reinforcement to the understanding of persistent pain behavior. The model assumes a priori that pain behaviors are maintained by reinforcing stimuli. However, the mere availability of environmental stimuli that are potential reinforcers does not establish a functional relationship between the behavior and the reward. The control of a stimulus over the behavior that precedes it must be demonstrated experimentally, and this has not been empirically established by operant pain studies in the analysis of the frequency of pain behaviors (Jaynes 1985). In addition, the operant pain literature seems to imply that behavior in all chronic pain patients is exclusively reinforced only by the promise of money and attention or the opportunity for avoidance. But reinforcers differ across individuals and are linked to an associated level of deprivation (Skinner 1953). Operant theory would predict, for example, that social attention should be a more potent reinforcer for a socially isolated (and deprived) pain patient than for one with plentiful social support. Operant pain theory has neglected to consider the issue of associated level of deprivation when examining the nature of reinforcement of pain behavior.

Moreover, the myopic attention to reinforcement specific to pain behaviors fails to consider the patient's entire repertoire and the effect of persistent pain in altering functional relationships between nonpain behaviors and reinforcement. The downside of chronic pain, with its associated disruption of income, social role, social support, self-worth, recreation, and work status, has been described as *secondary losses* (Fishbain 1994). This term reflects, on balance, the pervasive diminution of reinforcement in the life of a chronic pain patient and raises questions about the relative value of pain behavior–induced rewards in the context of the wide array of available reinforcers (Epstein 1992). In addition, stimuli that were premorbidly associated with high-frequency behaviors for many chronic pain patients, such as work (Blumer and Heilbronn 1982; Gamsa and Vikis-Freibergs 1991), and thus were presumably reinforcing, become for the operant pain model a source of aversion (e.g., presumed work avoidance). The model does not adequately address how, under these circumstances, a reinforcing stimulus condition transforms its functional relationship to the same behavior.

Data from clinical studies also raise questions about the operant nature of chronic pain. Pain behavior rather than pain experience is said to be amenable to operant mechanisms, but studies have reported a significant association between pain behavior and pain intensity (Romano et al. 1988). Also contrary to operant pain theory, patients receiving as-needed administration of analgesics during pain treatment are able to successfully reduce their use of medications while increasing their function (Keefe et al. 1981). Furthermore, evidence from observational studies indicates a positive relationship between pain behaviors and number of surgeries, abnormal physical findings, and depression (Keefe and Block 1982; Keefe et al. 1984, 1986), suggesting that factors beyond reinforcement (e.g., pain) may account for pain behaviors.

Major interest in the effect of reinforcement on pain behaviors has focused on both the marital interaction of chronic pain couples (Turk et al. 1987) and the effect of pending litigation or compensation on accident-related pain disability (Shapiro and Roth 1993). Consistent with operant theory, several observational studies have shown a relationship between the solicitousness of spouse responses and increased patient pain behavior (Block et al. 1980; Romano et al. 1995). Chronic pain patients who perceive their spouse as positively attentive to their pain report higher levels of functional disability (Kerns et al. 1991). However, these relationships appear to hold only for men (Flor et al. 1989) and may represent a reduction in adaptive coping when a spouse is present rather than the operation of reinforcement (Flor et al. 1995a). Turk and colleagues (Kerns et al. 1990; Turk et al. 1992) reported and replicated the important finding that spouse solicitousness and patient pain reports are significantly associated but only for couples who describe their marriage as highly satisfying. The authors concluded that cognitive variables such as the patient's appraisal of the quality of the marital relationship appear to mediate the effect of spousal response on pain behavior.

Studies of social support among chronic pain patients similarly questioned the linear nature of spousal attentiveness and pain disability. Gil et al. (1987) assessed indices of social support for a group of chronic pain patients. The perception of high satisfaction with, but not degree of availability of, social support was associated with a greater number of pain behaviors. Curiously, the authors interpreted these findings in support of an operant model, although presumably the density rather than the quality of social reward would be considered more pertinent to reinforcement potential. Conversely, other studies have reported a positive association between social support and decreased pain and disability (Jamison and Virts 1990), more adaptive coping with pain (Manne and Zautra 1989), and less depression (Goldberg et al. 1993). In addition, pain treatment studies that specifically examined the effects of interventions that address spousal attention to pain behavior had disappointing findings (Radojevic et al. 1992).

The literature pertaining to the effects of litigation and compensation factors on chronic pain disability is vast, and an adequate review is beyond the scope of this chapter. Since the influential writings of Miller (1961), it has become convention to assume that a chronic pain patient who has a pending claim or who is receiving pain-related compensation will remain disabled as long as the promise of reward is evident. Operant enthusiasts have repeatedly appealed to the monetary incentives associated with compensable injury as an explanation for persistent pain behavior (Weintraub 1992). However, a prudent and balanced scrutiny of available empirical studies did not identify a primary relationship between financial remuneration or its promise and various indices of pain disability (Mendelson 1986; Shapiro and Roth 1993). In many litigants who have pain from a compensable injury, pain symptoms improve and normal function returns before settlement (Schofferman and Wasserman 1994). Gallagher et al. (1995) reported that the availability of compensation had no appreciable effect on return to work rates for chronic low back pain patients after pain rehabilitation. In addition, chronic pain patients continue to experience significant pain, psychosocial distress, and disability despite settlement of their claims (Blanchard et al. 1998; Talo et al. 1989). Moreover, several authors have proposed that the exaggerated pain behavior and psychological disturbance observed among many chronic pain litigants might actually result from the stresses of the medicolegal system rather than the motive of avarice (Guest and Drummond 1992; J. Walker et al. 1999).

In summary, the operant model of chronic pain appears to have had a pervasive influence on the conceptualization and treatment of chronic pain despite serious flaws in theory and equivocal experimental findings. Some chronic pain patients are definitely motivated by secondary gain factors, whether they involve the pursuit of monetary reward or the avoidance of perceived aversive life situations. However, the wholesale presumption of secondary reward as an explanation of chronic pain and disability is not warranted by the available data. The successful treatment of chronic pain disability by operant methods is not sufficient to establish that the etiology of pain behavior is operantly conditioned (Jaynes 1985; Linton and G'otestam 1985). The focus on pain behavior rather than pain experience, and the attribution of pain expression to environmental factors, has diverted attention away from alternative and more inclusive models of chronic pain (e.g., cognitive-behavioral) (Novy et al. 1995; Turk and Flor 1987). Its effect also has been experienced by the many incredulous chronic pain patients who seek resolution of their private suffering and are informed that the answer resides in the environment.

Summary

It is ironic that as basic pain research has unraveled the intricacies and complexities of chronic pain physiology, for many clinicians, the practice of pain medicine has turned increasingly to nonspecific and univariate psychological models of pain causation. The lag of pain practice behind pain science rests on the former's overarching reliance on two outmoded assumptions in interpreting clinical chronic pain: the dualism of mind-body and the classic peripheralist view of sensorineural pain activation. Both of these anachronistic perspectives are undermined by the fact that pain differs from pure sensory phenomena by virtue of its inherent adhesion to affect. Thus, the indivisible link of sensation with affect in the perception of pain renders moot the consideration of one (affect) as a sole cause of the other (pain sensation) as a general principle of pain causation.

In this review, I have critically examined the theoretical basis and empirical support for three proposed psychological models of chronic pain and concluded that, as a generally applicable formulation, each model is inadequate. In select cases, each paradigm has relevance, as any pain clinician will testify. The exact frequency of psychodynamic, depression-induced, and operant pain is unknown. Obvious and serious methodological problems prevent determination of these prevalence rates. These data are important, however, because clinical decision making in pain assessment should focus on probability estimates of psychogenic pain. Unfortunately, in the absence of such information, errors in decision making can result when a patient with chronic pain is evaluated. For example, the prominence of psychological disturbance or the saliency that attends the frustrating treatment of a "difficult" pain patient can contribute to examiner bias in overestimating the probability of psychogenic pain among the chronic pain population (Dawson and Arkes 1987).

It is past due for pain clinicians to adopt a multivariate perspective of chronic pain and its related morbidity. Chronic pain has been treated too often as a distinct syndrome with common clinical characteristics and treatment needs (Turk 1990). The psychodynamic, depression variant, and operant models of chronic pain share this homogeneity assumption. Such univariate paradigms distract investigators from considering alternative mechanisms of pain disability (Turk and Flor 1987) and, by implication, encourage generic treatment options for vast numbers of chronic pain patients. Many patients have failed to benefit from intervention within this clinical framework (Turk 1990).

A biopsychosocial model offers a blueprint for the future of pain medicine. While seemingly overinclusive and broad, this model emphasizes the multifactorial and systems nature of clinical pain that is compatible with the accumulating data from laboratory and clinical studies. As such, it draws attention to interactional processes and mediating variables in elucidating the parameters of chronic pain. For example, recent evidence suggests that the nature of pain onset, if traumatically induced and resulting in posttraumatic stress symptoms, interacts with clinical variables to help explain the more severe affective distress and disability frequently observed among accident-related (and compensable) pain (Geisser et al. 1996). A second example derives from the literature on the role of cognitive appraisals in mediating pain disability. Cognitive variables such as pain beliefs, catastrophizing, and perceived control have been shown to mediate (and account for) the apparent associations between pain and its attendant disability and depression (Banks and Kerns 1996; Geisser and Roth 1998). These data illustrate the need for multivariate models in the conceptualization of chronic pain, with the hope that patient satisfaction will be the simple result.

References

Adler RH, Zlot S, Hurny C, et al: Engel's "psychogenic pain and the pain-prone patient": a retrospective, controlled clinical study. Psychosom Med 51:87–101, 1989

Affleck G, Tennen H, Urrows S, et al: Neuroticism and the pain-mood relation in rheumatoid arthritis: insights from a prospective daily study. J Consult Clin Psychol 60:119–126, 1992

American Psychiatric Association: Diagnostic and Statistical Manual of Mental Disorders, 3rd Edition. Washington, DC, American Psychiatric Association, 1980

American Psychiatric Association: Diagnostic and Statistical Manual of Mental Disorders, 3rd Edition, Revised. Washington, DC, American Psychiatric Association, 1987

American Psychiatric Association: Diagnostic and Statistical Manual of Mental Disorders, 4th Edition. Washington, DC, American Psychiatric Association, 1994

Anderson TP, Cole TM, Gullickson G, et al: Behavior modification of chronic pain: a treatment program by a multidisciplinary team. Clin Orthop 129:96–100, 1977

Andersson HI, Ejlertsson G, Leden I, et al: Chronic pain in a geographically defined general population: studies of differences in age, gender, social class, and pain lateralization. Clin J Pain 9:174–182, 1993

Atkinson JH, Slater MA, Patterson TL, et al: Prevalence, onset, and risk of psychiatric disorders in men with chronic low back pain. Pain 45:111–121, 1991

Atkinson JH, Slater MA, Williams RA, et al: A placebo-controlled randomized clinical trial of nortriptyline for chronic low back pain. Pain 76:287–296, 1998

Averill PM, Novy DM, Nelson DV, et al: Correlates of depression in chronic pain patients: a comprehensive examination. Pain 65:93–100, 1996

Awerbuch MS: Whiplash in Australia: illness or injury? Med J Aust 157:193–196, 1992

Badley EM, Rasooly I, Webster GK: Relative importance of musculoskeletal disorders as a cause of chronic health problems, disability, and health care utilization: findings from the Ontario health survey. J Rheumatol 21:505–514, 1994

Banks SM, Kerns RD: Explaining high rates of depression in chronic pain: a diathesis-stress formulation. Psychol Bull 119:95–110, 1996

Basbaum AI, Moss MS, Glazer EJ: Opiate and stimulation-produced analgesia: the contribution of the monoamines, in Advances in Pain Research and Therapy, Vol 5. Edited by Bonica JJ. New York, Raven, 1983, pp 323–339

Beard RW, Highman JW, Pearce S, et al: Diagnosis of pelvic varicosities in women with chronic pelvic pain. Lancet ii:946–949, 1984

Bendtsen L, Jensen R, Olesen J: Qualitatively altered nociception in chronic myofascial pain. Pain 65:259–264, 1996

Beutler LE, Engle D, Oro'Beutler ME, et al: Inability to express intense affect: a common link between depression and pain. J Consult Clin Psychol 54:752–759, 1986

Blanchard EB, Andrasik F, Neff D, et al: Biofeedback and relaxation training with three kinds of headache: treatment effects and their prediction. J Consult Clin Psychol 50:562–575, 1982

Blanchard EB, Hickling EJ, Taylor AE, et al: Effects of litigation settlements on posttraumatic stress symptoms in motor vehicle accident victims. J Trauma Stress 11:337–354, 1998

Blazer DG: Narcissism and the development of chronic pain. Int J Psychiatr Med 10:69–77, 1980–81

Block AR, Kremer EF, Gaylor M: Behavioral treatment of chronic pain: the wife as a discriminative cue for pain behavior. Pain 9:243–252, 1980

Blumer D, Heilbronn M: Chronic pain as a variant of depressive disease: the pain-prone disorder. J Nerv Ment Dis 170:381–406, 1982

Blumer D, Zorick F, Heilbronn M, et al: Biological markers for depression in chronic pain. J Nerv Ment Dis 170:425–428, 1982

Bonica JJ: Management of myofascial pain syndromes in general practice. JAMA 164:732–738, 1957

Bonica JJ, Sola AE: Other painful disorders of the low back, in The Management of Pain, 2nd Edition. Edited by Bonica JJ. Philadelphia, PA, Lea & Febiger, 1992, pp 1484–1514

Briere J, Runtz M: The long-term effects of sexual abuse: a review and hypothesis. New Dir Ment Health Serv 51:3–13, 1991

Calliet R: Chronic pain: is it necessary? Arch Phys Med Rehabil 60:4–7, 1979

Cherkin DC, Deyo RA, Street JH, et al: Predicting poor outcomes for back pain seen in primary care using patients' own criteria. Spine 21:2900–2907, 1996

Coderre TJ, Katz J, Vaccarino AL, et al: Contribution of central neuroplasticity to pathological pain: review of clinical and experimental evidence. Pain 52:259–285, 1993

Cohen MR, Pickar D, Extein I, et al: Plasma cortisol and B-endorphin immunoreactivity in nonmajor and major depression. Am J Psychiatry 141:628–632, 1984

Cox GB, Chapman CR, Black RG: The MMPI and chronic pain: the diagnosis of psychogenic pain. J Behav Med 1:437–443, 1978

Crofford LJ, Pillemar SR, Kalogeras KT, et al: Hypothalamic-pituitary-adrenal axis perturbations in patients with fibromyalgia. Arthritis Rheum 37:1583–1592, 1994

Crook J, Tunks E, Rideout E, et al: Epidemiologic comparison of persistent pain sufferers in a specialty pain clinic and in the community. Arch Phys Med Rehabil 67:451–455, 1986

Dawson NV, Arkes HR: Systematic errors in medical decision making: judgment limitations. J Gen Intern Med 2:183–187, 1987

Deyo RA: Accuracy of the history and physical examination for detecting clinically important lumbar disc herniations, in Low Back Pain: A Scientific and Clinical Overview. Edited by Weinstein SW, Gordon SL. Rosemont, IL, American Academy of Orthopaedic Surgeons, 1996, pp 61–71

Duncan GH, Bushnell MC, Bates R, et al: Task related responses of monkey medullary dorsal horn neurones. J Neurophysiol 57:289–310, 1987

Durrani Z, Winnie AP: Piriformis muscle syndrome: an underdiagnosed cause of sciatica. J Pain Symptom Manage 6:374–379, 1991

Dworkin RH, Caligor E: Psychiatric diagnosis and chronic pain: DSM-III-R and beyond. J Pain Symptom Manage 3:87–98, 1988

Dworkin RH, Richlin DM, Handlin DS, et al: Predicting treatment response in depressed and non-depressed chronic pain patients. Pain 24:343–353, 1986

Engel GL: "Psychogenic" pain and the pain-prone patient. Am J Med 26:899–918, 1959

Engels M-L, Moisan D, Harris R: MMPI indices of childhood trauma among 110 female outpatients. J Pers Assess 63:135–147, 1994

Epstein LH: Role of behavior theory in behavioral medicine. J Consult Clin Psychol 60:493–498, 1992

Faucett JA: Depression in painful chronic disorders: the role of pain and conflict about pain. J Pain Symptom Manage 9:520–526, 1994

Feinmann C: Pain relief by antidepressants: possible modes of action. Pain 23:1–8, 1985

Fields HL, Basbaum AI: Endogenous pain control mechanisms, in Textbook of Pain, 3rd Edition. Edited by Wall PD, Melzack R. London, Churchill Livingstone, 1994, pp 206–217

Fishbain DA: Secondary gain concept: definition problems and its abuse in medical practice. American Pain Society Journal 3:264–273, 1994

Fishbain DA, Goldberg M, Meagher RB, et al: Male and female chronic pain patients categorized by DSM-III psychiatric diagnostic criteria. Pain 26:181–197, 1986

Fishbain DA, Cutler RB, Rosomoff HL, et al: Chronic pain-associated depression: antecedent or consequence of chronic pain: a review. Clin J Pain 13:116–137, 1997

Fishbain DA, Cutler RB, Rosomoff HL, et al: Comorbidity between psychiatric disorders and chronic pain. Current Review of Pain 2:1–10, 1998a

Fishbain DA, Cutler RB, Rosomoff HL, et al: Do antidepressants have an analgesic effect in psychogenic pain and somatoform pain disorder? a meta-analysis. Psychosom Med 60:503–509, 1998b

Flor H, Turk DC, Rudy TE: Relationship of pain impact and significant other reinforcement of pain behaviors: the mediating role of gender, marital status, and marital satisfaction. Pain 38:45–50, 1989

Flor H, Breitenstein C, Birbaumer N, et al: A psychophysiologic analysis of spouse solicitousness towards pain behaviors, spouse interaction, and pain perception. Behavior Therapy 26:255–272, 1995a

Flor H, Elbert T, Knecht S, et al: Phantom-limb pain as a perceptual correlate of cortical reorganization following arm amputation. Nature 375:482–484, 1995b

Fordyce WE: Behavioral Methods for Chronic Pain and Illness. St. Louis, MO, Mosby, 1976

Fordyce WE: Environmental factors in the genesis of low back pain, in Advances in Pain Research and Therapy, Vol 3. Edited by Bonica JJ, Liebeskind JC, Albe-Fessard DG. New York, Raven, 1979, pp 659–666

Fordyce WE (ed): Back Pain in the Workplace: Management of Disability in Non-Specific Conditions. Seattle, WA, IASP Press, 1995

Fordyce WE, Fowler RS, Lehman JF, et al: Operant conditioning in the treatment of chronic pain. Arch Phys Med Rehabil 54:399–408, 1973

Fordyce WE, Shelton JL, Dundore DE: The modification of avoidance learning pain behaviors. J Behav Med 5:405–414, 1982

France RD, Krishnan KRR, Houpt JL, et al: Differentiation of depression from chronic pain with the dexamethasone suppression test and DSM-III. Am J Psychiatry 141:1577–1579, 1984

Freud S: New Introductory Lectures on Psychoanalysis, 2nd Edition, Vol 24. London, Hogarth Press, 1937

Gallagher RM: Secondary gain in pain medicine: let us stick with biobehavioral data. American Pain Society Journal 3:274–278, 1994

Gallagher RM: The complex relationship between pain and depression. Current Review of Pain 3:24–41, 1999

Gallagher RM, Myers P: Referral delay in back pain patients on worker's compensation: costs and policy implications. Psychosomatics 37:270–284, 1996

Gallagher RM, Williams RA, Skelly J, et al: Workers' compensation and return-to-work in low back pain. Pain 61:299–307, 1995

Gamsa A: Is emotional disturbance a precipitator or a consequence of chronic pain? Pain 42:183–195, 1990

Gamsa A: The role of psychological factors in chronic pain, I: a half century of study. Pain 57:5–15, 1994

Gamsa A, Vikis-Freibergs V: Psychological events are both risk factors in and consequences of chronic pain. Pain 44:271–277, 1991

Geisser ME, Roth RS: Knowledge of and agreement with chronic pain diagnoses: relation to affective distress, pain beliefs and coping, pain intensity and disability. Journal of Occupational Rehabilitation 8:73–88, 1998

Geisser ME, Roth RS, Bachman JE, et al: The relationship between symptoms of post-traumatic stress disorder and pain, affective disturbance and disability among patients with accident and non-accident related pain. Pain 66:207–214, 1996

Geisser ME, Roth RS, Robinson ME: Assessing depression among persons with chronic pain using the Center of Epidemiological Studies—Depression Scale and the Beck Depression Inventory: a comparative analysis. Clin J Pain 13:163–170, 1997

Gil KM, Keefe FJ, Crisson JE, et al: Social support and pain behavior. Pain 29:209–217, 1987

Goldberg GM, Kerns RD, Rosenberg R: Pain-relevant support as a buffer from depression among chronic pain patients low in instrumental activity. Clin J Pain 9:34–40, 1993

Gracely RH, Lynch SA, Bennett GJ: Painful neuropathy: altered central processing maintained dynamically by peripheral input. Pain 51:175–194, 1992

Graff-Radford SB, Jaeger B, Reeves JL: Myofascial pain may present clinically as occipital neuralgia. Neurosurgery 19:610–613, 1986

Greenman PE: Principles of Manual Medicine, 2nd Edition. Baltimore, MD, Williams & Wilkins, 1996

Guest GH, Drummond PD: Effect of compensation on emotional state and disability in chronic back pain. Pain 48:125–130, 1992

Haddox JD: Appropriate use of the chronic pain specialist and the role of conceptual fluidity, in Pain Treatment Centers at a Crossroads: A Practical and Conceptual Reappraisal. Edited by Cohen MJM, Campbell JN. Seattle, WA, IASP Press, 1996, pp 297–306

Haythornthwaite JA, Sieber WJ, Kerns RD: Depression and the chronic pain experience. Pain 46:177–184, 1991

Heinrich RL, Cohen MJ, Naliboff BD, et al: Comparing physical and behavior therapy for chronic low back pain on physical abilities, psychological distress, and patients' perceptions. J Behav Med 8:61–78, 1985

Hendler NH, Kozikowski JG: Overlooked physical diagnoses in chronic pain patients involved in litigation. Psychosomatics 34:494–501, 1993

Jamison RN, Virts KL: The influence of family support on chronic pain. Behav Res Ther 28:283–287, 1990

Janda V: Muscles and motor control in cervicogenic pain syndromes: assessment and management, in Physical Therapy of the Cervical and Thoracic Spine. Edited by Grand R. New York, Churchill Livingstone, 1994, pp 195–216

Jaynes J: Sensory pain and conscious pain. Behav Brain Sci 8:61–63, 1985

Jensen MP, Turner JA, Romano JM, et al: Coping with chronic pain: a critical review of the literature. Pain 47:249–283, 1991

Jung AC, Staiger T, Sullivan M: The efficacy of selective serotonin reuptake inhibitors for the management of chronic pain. J Gen Intern Med 12:384–389, 1997

Katon W, Egan K, Miller D: Chronic pain: lifetime psychiatric diagnoses and family history. Am J Psychiatry 142:1156–1160, 1985

Keefe FJ, Block AR: Development of an observation method for assessing pain behavior in chronic low back pain patients. Behavior Therapy 13:363–375, 1982

Keefe FJ, Block AR, Williams RB, et al: Behavioral treatment of chronic low back pain: clinical outcome and individual differences in pain relief. Pain 11:221–231, 1981

Keefe FJ, Wilkins RH, Cook WA: Direct observation of pain behavior in low back pain patients during physical examination. Pain 20:59–68, 1984

Keefe FJ, Wilkins RH, Cook WA, et al: Depression, pain, and pain behavior. J Consult Clin Psychol 54:341–351, 1986

Kerns RD, Haythornthwaite J: Depression among chronic pain patients: cognitive-behavioral analysis and effect on rehabilitation outcome. J Consult Clin Psychol 56:870–876, 1988

Kerns RD, Haythornthwaite J, Southwick S, et al: The role of marital interaction in chronic pain and depressive symptom severity. J Psychosom Res 34:401–408, 1990

Kerns RD, Southwick S, Giller EL, et al: The relationship between reports of pain-related social interactions and expressions of pain and affective distress. Behavior Therapy 22:101–111, 1991

King SA: Review: DSM-IV and pain. Clin J Pain 11:171–176, 1995

Lacey H: Pain behavior: how to define this operant. Behav Brain Sci 8:64–65, 1985

Latimer PR: External contingency management for chronic pain: critical review of the evidence. Am J Psychiatry 10:1308–1312, 1982

Lautenbacher S, Roscher S, Strain D: Pain perception in depression: relationships to symptomatology and naloxone-sensitive mechanisms. Psychosom Med 56:345–352, 1994

Levine JD, Gordon NC, Smith R, et al: Desipramine enhances opiate post-operative analgesia. Pain 27:45–49, 1986

Linton SJ, G'otestam KG: Controlling pain reports through operant conditioning. Percept Mot Skills 60:427–437, 1985

Loeser JD: What is pain? Theoretical Medicine 12:213–225, 1991

Magni G, Moreschi C, Rigatti-Luchini S, et al: Prospective study on the relationship between depressive symptoms and chronic musculo-skeletal pain. Pain 56:289–297, 1994

Manne SL, Zautra AJ: Spouse criticism and support: their association with coping and psychological adjustment among women with rheumatoid arthritis. J Pers Soc Psychol 56:608–617, 1989

Maruta T, Vatterott MK, McHardy MJ: Pain management as an antidepressant: long-term resolution of pain-associated depression. Pain 36:335–337, 1989

Max MB: Antidepressant drugs, a treatment for chronic pain: efficacy and mechanisms, in Pain and the Brain: From Nociception to Cognition. Edited by Bromm B, Desmedt JE. New York, Raven, 1995, pp 510–515

Max MB, Culnane M, Schafer SC, et al: Amitriptyline relieves diabetic neuropathy pain in patients with normal and depressed mood. Neurology 37:589–596, 1987

Mechanic D: The concept of illness behavior. Journal of Chronic Diseases 15:189–194, 1962

Melzack R, Wall PD: Pain mechanisms: a new theory. Science 150:971–979, 1965

Mendelson G: Chronic pain and compensation: a review. J Pain Symptom Manage 1:135–144, 1986

Mense S: Referral of muscle pain: new aspects. American Pain Society Journal 3:1–9, 1994

Merskey H, Bogduk N: Classification of Chronic Pain: Description of Chronic Pain Syndromes and Definition of Pain Terms. Seattle, WA, IASP Press, 1994

Merskey H, Lau CL, Russell ES, et al: Screening for psychiatric morbidity: the pattern of psychological illness and premorbid characteristics in four chronic pain populations. Pain 330:141–157, 1987

Miller H: Accident neurosis. BMJ 1:919–925, 992–998, 1961

Niv D, Devor M: Preemptive analgesia in the relief of postoperative pain. Current Review of Pain 1:79–94, 1996

Novy DM, Nelson DV, Francis DJ, et al: Perspectives of chronic pain: an evaluative comparison of restrictive and comprehensive models. Psychol Bull 118:238–247, 1995

Onghena P, Van Houdenhove B. Antidepressant-induced analgesia in chronic non-malignant pain: a meta-analysis of 39 placebo-controlled studies. Pain 49:205–209, 1992

Owen-Salters E, Gatchel RJ, Polatin PB, et al: Changes in psychopathology following functional restoration of chronic low back pain: a prospective study. Journal of Occupational Rehabilitation 6:215–223, 1996

Pilowsky I: Pain as abnormal illness behavior. Journal of Human Stress 4:22–27, 1978

Punch MR, Roth RS, Pominville L: Musculoskeletal origins of chronic pelvic pain in women. Paper presented at the annual meeting of the American Society of Psychosomatic Obstetrics and Gynecology, San Diego, CA, February 1994

Radojevic V, Nicassio PM, Weisman MH: Behavioral intervention with and without family support in rheumatoid arthritis. Behavior Therapy 23:13–30, 1992

Ranaer M, Vertommen H, Nijs P, et al: Chronic pelvic pain without obvious pathology in women. Eur J Obstet Gynecol Reprod Biol 10:415–463, 1980

Rapkin AJ, Kames LD, Darke LL, et al: History of physical and sexual abuse in women with chronic pelvic pain. Obstet Gynecol 76:92–96, 1990

Reich I, Rosenblatt RM, Tupin J: DSM-III: a new nomenclature for classifying patients with chronic pain. Pain 16:201–206, 1983

Reid J, Ewan C, Lowy E: Pilgrimage of pain: the illness experience of women with repetition strain injury and the search for credibility. Soc Sci Med 32:601–612, 1991

Reiter RC, Shakarin LR, Gambone JC, et al: Correlation between sexual abuse and somatization in women with somatic and nonsomatic chronic pelvic pain. Am J Obstet Gynecol 165:104–109, 1991

Reynolds DB: Surgery in the rat during electrical analgesia induced by focal brain stimulation. Science 164:444–445, 1969

Rind B, Tromovich P, Bauserman R: A meta-analytic examination of assumed properties of child sexual abuse using college samples. Psychol Bull 124:22–53, 1998

Roberts A, Reinhardt L: The behavioral management of chronic pain: long-term follow-up with comparison groups. Pain 5:151–162, 1980

Romano JM, Turner JA: Chronic pain and depression: does the evidence support a relationship? Psychol Bull 97:18–34, 1985

Romano JM, Syrjala KL, Levy RL: Overt pain behaviors: relationship to patient functioning and treatment outcome. Behavior Therapy 19.191–201, 1988

Romano JM, Turner JA, Jensen MP, et al: Chronic pain patient-spouse behavioral interactions predict pain disability. Pain 63:353–360, 1995

Rosomoff HL, Fishbain DA, Goldberg M, et al: Physical findings in patients with chronic intractable benign pain of the back and/or neck. Pain 37:279–287, 1989

Roth RS, Horowitz KE, Bachman JE: Chronic myofascial pain: knowledge of diagnosis and satisfaction with treatment. Arch Phys Med Rehabil 79:966–970, 1998

Roy R: Engel's pain-prone disorder patient: 25 years after. Psychother Psychosom 43:126–135, 1985

Salovey P, Birnbaum D: Influence of mood on health-relevant cognitions. J Pers Soc Psychol 57:539–551, 1989

Schmidt AJM: The behavioral management of pain: a criticism of a response. Pain 30:285–291, 1987

Schmidt AJM, Gierlings REH, Peters ML: Environmental and interoceptive influences on chronic low back pain. Pain 38:137–143, 1989

Schofferman J, Wasserman S: Successful treatment of low back pain and neck pain after a motor vehicle accident despite litigation. Spine 19:1007–1010, 1994

Shapiro AP, Roth RS: The effect of litigation on recovery from whiplash, in Spine: State of the Art Reviews: Cervical Flexion-Extension/Whiplash Injuries. Edited by Teasell RW, Shapiro AP. Philadelphia, PA, Hanley & Belfus, 1993, pp 531–556

Shapiro AP, Teasell RW: Misdiagnosis and chronic pain as hysteria and malingering. Current Review of Pain 2:19–28, 1998

Simons DG, Travell JG, Simons LS: Myofascial Pain and Dysfunction: The Trigger Point Manual, Vol 1. Baltimore, MD, Williams & Wilkins, 1999

Skinner BF: The generic nature of the concepts of stimulus and response. J Gen Psychol 12:40–65, 1935

Skinner BF: Science and Human Behavior. New York, Macmillan, 1953

Stratton-Hill C Jr: When will adequate pain treatment be the norm? JAMA 274:1881–1882, 1995

Sullivan MJL, Reesor K, Mikail S, et al: The treatment of depression in chronic low back pain: review and recommendations. Pain 50:5–13, 1992

Talo S, Hendler N, Brodie J: Effects of active and completed litigation on treatment results: worker's compensation patients compared with other litigation patients. Journal of Occupational Medicine 31:265–269, 1989

Tauschke E, Merskey H, Helmes E: Psychological defense mechanisms in patients with pain. Pain 40:161–170, 1990

Tinling DC, Klein RF: Psychogenic pain and aggression: the syndrome of the solitary hunter. Psychosom Med 28:738–748, 1966

Travell JG: Identification of myofascial trigger point syndromes: a case of atypical neuralgia. Arch Phys Med Rehabil 62:100–106, 1981

Turk DC: Customizing treatment for chronic pain patients: who, what, and why. Clin J Pain 6:250–270, 1990

Turk DC, Flor H: Etiological theories and treatment for chronic back pain, II: psychological models and interventions. Pain 19:209–233, 1984

Turk DC, Flor H: Pain>pain behaviors: the utility and limitations of the pain behavior construct. Pain 31:277–295, 1987

Turk DC, Salovey P: "Chronic pain as a variant of depressive disease": a critical reappraisal. J Nerv Ment Dis 172:398–404, 1984

Turk DC, Flor H, Rudy TE: Pain and families, I: etiology, maintenance, and psychosocial impact. Pain 30:3–27, 1987

Turk DC, Kerns RD, Rosenberg R: Effects of marital interaction on chronic pain and disability: examining the downside. Rehabilitation Psychology 37:259–274, 1992

Turkington RW: Depression masquerading as diabetic neuropathy. JAMA 243:1147–1150, 1980

Turner JA, Chapman CR: Psychological interventions for chronic pain: a critical review, II: operant conditioning, hypnosis, and cognitive-behavior therapy. Pain 12:23–46, 1982

Turner JA, Clancy S, McQuade KJ, et al: Effectiveness of behavioral therapy for chronic low back pain. J Consult Clin Psychol 58:573–579, 1990

Van Houdenhove B: Prevalence and psychodynamic interpretation of premorbid hyperactivity in patients with chronic pain. Psychother Psychosom 45:195–200, 1986

Violon A: Family etiology of chronic pain. International Journal of Family Therapy 7:235–246, 1985

Von Knorring L, Perris C, Eisemann M, et al: Pain as a symptom of depressive disorders, I: relationship to diagnostic subgroup and depressive symptomatology. Pain 15:19–26, 1983

Von Korff M, LeResche L, Dworkin SF: First onset of common pain symptoms: a prospective study of depression as a risk factor. Pain 55:251–258, 1993

Waddell G: Low back disability. Neurosurg Clin N Am 2:719–737, 1991

Waddell G: Low back pain: a twentieth century health care enigma. Spine 21:2820–2825, 1996

Waddell G, McCullough JA, Kummel E, et al: Nonorganic physical signs in low back pain. Spine 5:117–125, 1989

Wade JB, Dougherty LM, Hart RP, et al: Patterns of normal personality structure among chronic pain patients. Pain 48:37–43, 1992

Walker EA, Katon W, Harrop-Griffiths J, et al: Relationship of chronic pelvic pain to psychiatric diagnoses and childhood sexual abuse. Am J Psychiatry 145:75–80, 1988

Walker EA, Sullivan MD, Stenchever MA: Use of antidepressants in the management of women with chronic pelvic pain. Obstet Gynecol Clin North Am 20:743–751, 1993

Walker EA, Keegan D, Gardner G, et al: Psychosocial factors in fibromyalgia compared with rheumatoid arthritis, II: sexual, physical and emotional abuse and neglect. Psychosom Med 59:572–577, 1997

Walker J, Holloway I, Sofaer B: In the system: the lived experience of chronic back pain from the perspective of those seeking help from pain clinics. Pain 80:621–628, 1999

Wall PD: Introduction to the edition after this one, in Textbook of Pain, 3rd Edition. Edited by Wall PD, Melzack R. London, Churchill Livingstone, 1994, pp 1–7

Ward NG, Bloom VL, Friedel RO: The effectiveness of tricyclic antidepressants in the treatment of coexisting pain and depression. Pain 7:331–341, 1979

Watkins LR, Mayer DJ: Organization of endogenous opiates and non-opiate pain control systems. Science 216:1185–1192, 1982

Weinreb JC, Wolbarscht LB, Cohen JM, et al: Prevalence of lumbosacral intervertebral disc abnormalities on MR images in pregnant and asymptomatic non-pregnant women. Radiology 172:125–128, 1989

Weintraub MI: Regional pain is usually hysterical. Arch Neurol 45:914–915, 1988

Weintraub MI: Litigation-chronic pain syndrome—a distinct entity: analysis of 210 cases. American Journal of Pain Management 2:198–204, 1992

Wells KB, Stewart A, Hays RD, et al: The functioning and well-being of depressed patients. JAMA 262:914–919, 1989

Ziesat HA, Angle H, Gentry WD, et al: Drug use and misuse in operant pain patients. Addict Behav 4:263–266, 1979

.

Chapter 4
Pain Rounds

The Experts Comment

Mary Jane Massie, M.D.
Lisa Chertkov, M.D.
Stewart B. Fleishman, M.D.
Barbara Kamholz, M.D.
Philip R. Muskin, M.D.
Randy S. Roth, Ph.D.

> There's a vicious and strong temptation to nurture the hurt we wail about. The hurting has so nearly become us—become the whole core of our present self—that the thought of finally dismissing it from us feels scarily like desertion or killing.
>
> *Reynolds Price[1]*

Patients with pain syndromes commonly present to psychiatrists. All too often, these patients are referred for psychiatric evaluation when all else has failed, in a last-ditch effort to put together all of the pieces, find an explanation for symptoms that have not adequately responded to treatment, and resolve complex, and often long-standing, interpersonal and family conflicts. Thus, it is not surprising that patients with chronic pain often have complex medical histories, and equally complex life histories, multiple pain problems, and comorbid psychiatric disorders. The referring doctor expects the psychiatric consultant to diagnose and manage the psychiatric symptoms, as well as shed light on the treatment of the patient's pain syndrome.

---

[1] Reprinted with the permission of Scribner's, a Division of Simon & Schuster Inc. from A WHOLE NEW LIFE by Reynolds Price. Copyright © 1994 Reynolds Price.

In the previous chapters of this monograph, pain syndromes are described, and guidelines for pharmacological and nonpharmacological treatments are outlined. In this chapter, the initial psychiatric consultations on four patients with chronic pain are presented, each approached from a different perspective by expert clinicians. The syndromes presented are those commonly seen in a psychiatrist's office: neuropathic pain, migraine headache, fibromyalgia, and chronic low back pain. The discussants in this case conference are a diverse group of clinicians (directors of pain clinics, consultation-liaison psychiatrists, psychoanalysts, and cognitive-behavioral psychologists who specialize in pain), each of whom brings a unique perspective to patient assessment and care.

These patients have complex and multifaceted problems. Our experts discuss their initial impressions of each patient and outline considerations for further evaluation, treatment, and difficulties that will likely be encountered during the psychiatric treatment of these patients. In this clinical case conference, our experts explore relevant issues in developing a diagnostic framework that incorporates medical and psychiatric symptoms as well as psychosocial variables, dealing with countertransference, forming a therapeutic alliance with a "treatment-refractory" patient, and negotiating family systems. Each expert clinician brings a unique perspective to patient evaluation and treatment; and, in combination, they provide a comprehensive approach to difficult pain syndromes.

Case 1: Recurrent Neuropathic Pain in an Elderly Woman With Suicidal Thinking

A 75-year-old, twice-divorced and now widowed, retired, successful psychologist is sent to you for evaluation by her internist. The internist states that "this lovely, energetic woman, who knows what she wants, had a right mastectomy and axillary dissection for breast cancer 7 years ago. All nodes were negative, she had no radiation or chemotherapy, and she has had no evidence of recurrence but now has neuropathic pain. Her previous psychiatrist recently retired and moved to another state." The internist notes that it is unclear whether this psychologically minded clinician needs psychotherapy, but he feels that she needs some kind of support because she has experienced multiple life losses.

Your new patient appears 10–15 years younger than her stated age. She is clearly intelligent, educated, sophisticated, and opinionated. However, she looks both distressed and in pain. She apologizes for not being as alert as she likes to be, attributing this to the drugs she is taking for pain: amitriptyline (35 mg at bedtime) and Percocet (1–2 tablets every 3 hours).

The patient's first episode of neuropathic pain occurred 2½ years ago; she has had two subsequent episodes, each 9–12 months apart. These episodes of severe, incapacitating pain have each lasted 3–4 months. Her first episode of pain was treated presumptively with acyclovir even though no herpetic lesions were seen. Her pain always starts under her left breast and extends around her chest to the left scapula. The pain is described as varying both in quality ("burning, stabbing, prickling") and in intensity. At the time of your visit with her, she states that her pain is about 3 on a 0- to 10-point scale, but in the past 2 days, she rated her pain as 7–9 and spent most of the day in bed because of it. The patient shows you her notebook in which she records the names and doses of her medications and rates her pain intensity when she takes the medications. She states that her last psychiatrist encouraged her to keep this pain diary, an exercise that has been useful to her because review of her diary helps her see that she has some "good days and fairly good days," during which time she can participate in some activities. Although retired, she works 5–40 hours per week as a volunteer research assistant and mentor for students who have recently graduated from her professional school. She actively visits the theater, movies, and museums. She states that after the death of her husband of 20 years, she has deliberately rekindled relationships with professional colleagues and former friends.

Consistent with the information provided by the referring physician, the patient describes a series of losses that have occurred in the last 4 years. Two friends, her younger brother, and her older sister have all died, as did her beloved third husband. She describes having been suicidal after the death of her husband and credits her previous psychiatrist with having helped her "reestablish a life" after his death. The patient is annoyed when you ask her to describe her history, stating that she has "worked through" much of her life during the Freudian analysis that she undertook in her 30s and again recently in the analytically oriented psychotherapy that she undertook with her last psychiatrist. She experiences her psychiatrist's retirement and move as an additional profound loss.

The patient describes herself as being very depressed but, ultimately, the only successful child of an affluent couple. She had a "privileged childhood" and was doted on by her "wise, philanthropic" father and ignored by her "stupid, silly" mother. After she graduated from a university, she married twice, both times to men who were "life failures." During her second marriage and after multiple infertility workups, she adopted a very troubled child and became an "overly devoted mother." She made a near-fatal suicide attempt by overdose when her child was 7 years old and recalls being enraged when she woke up in an intensive care unit and found that she was alive. She states that now she can admit to herself that her adopted daughter was a "high-functioning borderline" who cruelly and rudely abandoned her when she was given the diagnosis of breast cancer.

In addition to the above-mentioned losses, the patient is in the process of watching several of her similar-aged friends deteriorate both mentally and physically. When asked about current suicidal thoughts, she appears irritated and matter-of-factly states that she has "stockpiled enough medication to kill a small city," but she indicates that her worst fear is "doing it badly and becoming a vegetable." The patient is fully oriented, and her cognitive processes and memory are grossly intact. She repeatedly says, "I wish you could see me the way I really am." She describes being praised by all who know her for being effervescent and extraordinarily determined and capable. She appears to be in pain, uncomfortable, and sad. She is impatient and somewhat irritable. Her speech is articulate and goal-directed, and no psychotic thought process or content is evident. At the end of the hour, she says, "I am not really sure what you can do for me; I have had years of therapy, and I think I really understand my issues very well. There is nothing you or anyone else can do to bring back the people who were important to me. You and I both know that I can always kill myself; I probably will. However, I have already told you that I don't have any intention of doing that right now. All I really want from you are suggestions about how to treat my pain. I won't go to another pain clinic; they make you wait. Don't send me for those MRIs, X rays, and CT scans; they never show anything. I took Paxil, Sinequan, Klonopin, Xanax, and Ativan; none of them work for me, and they make me sleepy. And don't prescribe that paste for pain; it's disgusting."

Dr. Massie: Stewart B. Fleishman, M.D., an expert in psychiatric oncology and palliative care, will show how to use the multiaxial framework for conceptualizing the management of pain in patients with comorbid psychiatric illness.

Dr. Fleishman: This case represents a somewhat "usual" request of psychiatrists who work in large cancer centers. The referring internist knows that the patient needs some kind of support but is not sure exactly what kind or to whom the patient should be referred. The patient, however, has a very specific request: to obtain relief from a nagging pain problem in a setting that will be sensitive to the *way* in which the care is provided and to have the responsible clinician not be frightened by the obstacle of chronic suicidal risk.

Thinking through a complex clinical problem requires a framework, an approach to sorting out all the details. The standard DSM-IV multiaxial classification can serve this purpose (American Psychiatric Association 1994). The patient is obviously distressed by her recurring pain problem, which would certainly qualify her for an adjustment disorder with mixed anxiety and depressed mood on Axis I. Multiple losses are presented: her health (cancer); her youth and expectations of fertility; her trusted psychiatrist; her friends who have fallen ill; her third husband (with whom she shared a successful marriage); her two friends, brother, and sister who died; and the emotional support she had hoped to receive from her adopted daughter. Traits of a narcissistic personality disorder on Axis II color this patient's perceptions and her medical and personal relationships. Axis III is easily identified: node-negative breast cancer, NED (no evidence of disease), and postherpetic neuralgia. Axis IV shows severe psychosocial stressors, and Axis V shows a functional score of 85–90, indicating minimal functional impairment.

Obtain Treatment History

A successful treatment plan requires the doctor to work with the patient's need for control and her need to be treated more specially than the run-of-the-mill patient. Before considering new treatment strategies, the clinician should review pertinent records and do a thorough diagnostic evaluation, the first step of which is to obtain a detailed history of her symptoms and treatments:

- Breast cancer diagnostics (pathology reports of lesion and lymph node biopsies)
- Other treatments offered or given: chemotherapy, radiation therapy, hormonal therapy
- Tumor markers
- Reports of CT and MRI of the chest and bone scans at time of diagnosis and follow-up
- Recent chest X rays
- Recent blood work (complete blood count, hepatic and metabolic panels)

Utilize the DSM-IV Multiaxial System

Thereafter, the multiaxial system can provide a framework for considering further interventions and developing a strategic treatment plan.

The clinician should collect as much information as possible about previous pain management strategies, including medication trials (dosage and duration). Also, the patient should provide a complete list of all other medications, food supplements, vitamins, and herbs that she is taking or recently stopped taking.

Axis I: In treating an adjustment disorder, it is vital to acknowledge the distress that the patient is experiencing. Psychoeducation about healthy responses to life stresses and the identification and reinforcement of adaptive coping skills are often helpful. In addition, it will help to put her losses in the context of many "bad breaks" in the trajectory of her life as her strengths are reinforced. Cancer may evoke its own special terror and distress, but the patient's breast cancer has been diagnosed early and well treated and thus may be one of the most "fixable" of her problems. The pain problem may be somewhat less fixable, but several options can be tried before we reach that conclusion. Ruling out major depression, which could account for her suicidal feelings and pain, is a vital first step. However, assuming that one parsimonious diagnosis accounts for the total clinical picture will likely end up as an additional and unnecessary frustration for the patient, clinician, and other members of the treatment team, by erroneously pointing to a psychogenic cause for her pain.

Axis II: The patient's high standards for herself, her family, and her medical care should be reinforced and related to her current situation (being careful not to interpret her defenses or to break them down, which would have its place in dynamic long-term psychotherapy but not here and not now). The clinician should emphasize that the current suggestions to manage the pain problem are intended to be helpful and not to disappoint her. Her suicidal ideation should be discussed to verify the lack of intent and plan. The consultant should corroborate that her suicidal thoughts and plans are the last vestige of control that she has over her body and her life in general and that this dynamic is the fuel for these statements. Discussing her suicidal thoughts before a gesture and reviewing the legacy that suicide would leave on her extended family would be prudent, especially in view of her warehoused supply of medications.

Axis III: The consultant should reinforce the necessity of her pain diary and complement her on doing such a good job of keeping it (e.g., "This is one situation in which you can use your professional skills to help along your own care, the way you have done for countless others."). The addition of two other parameters for her diary, pain relief (0 = no relief, 10 = complete relief) and global quality of life (0 = worst, 10 = best), should be suggested so that treatment efficacy can be assessed, and the relation of treatment to a "good" day or "bad" day can be made. These tools reinforce the patient's active role in the treatment and provide valuable information for the assessment of the effect of her symptoms and the efficacy of any interventions.

Treatment Options

The clinician should explain the logic of the past and proposed treatment decisions. Categorizing the drugs used thus far is important in clarifying the mechanism of action and possible management strategies, as well as providing a framework to identify their effect on target symptoms:

- Tricyclic antidepressants (TCAs): amitriptyline (Elavil), doxepin (Sinequan)

- Selective serotonin reuptake inhibitors: paroxetine (Paxil)
- Benzodiazepines: alprazolam (Xanax), lorazepam (Ativan), clonazepam (Klonopin)
- Topical "anesthetic": capsaicin cream
- Opiate: acetaminophen with oxycodone (Percocet)

For each medication, the exact dosages used, length of the trial for each, and response to treatment should be determined.

- Substantiate that the patient has an understanding of the pathophysiology of herpetic infection and how it can result in nociceptive pain. Use analogies to electrical conduction if this will be meaningful to this patient.
- Indicate which drugs used thus far have a reliable track record of treating nociceptive pain (e.g., amitriptyline, doxepin, and clonazepam) and which drugs have less research to support their use (e.g., paroxetine) (Egbunike and Chaffee 1990).
- Explain the rationale for the use of anticonvulsants as analgesics and the concept of a therapeutic window (Swerdlow 1984). Describe the necessity of monitoring blood levels of some of these medications as a way to optimize treatment results. Because the patient has already expressed concern about the effects of her illness and symptoms on her quality of life, flexibility in scheduling phlebotomies to minimize inconvenience can be used as an example of the ways in which the patient can be empowered and her sense of control can be supported.
- Discuss alternatives: carbamazepine (Tegretol) or gabapentin (Neurontin) and the differences in the amount of sedation, hepatotoxicity, and effect on hematopoeisis expected from these drugs. Recommend gabapentin, which may be less sedating and offer a better quality of life. Some patients would expect your review of secondary options, such as diphenylhydantoin (Dilantin), valproic acid (Depakote), or lamotrigine (Lamictal), and your review of other off-label trials of dextromethorphan, various over-the-counter and prescription nonsteroidal anti-inflammatory drugs, oral anesthetics used as antiarrhythmics (such as mexiletine), or topical anesthetics (such as EMLA [eutectic mixture of local anesthetics]).

- Explain your plan to use single agents one at a time and then, if they are partially effective, to augment or to consider using two agents, with careful monitoring of blood levels. Remind your patient that these drugs have many interactions with other medications and that she should always check with the prescribing physician or her pharmacist when starting or stopping other medications. Also review the potential for food-drug interactions (e.g., grapefruit juice) (Rodvold and Meyer 1996).

Dr. Massie: Lisa Chertkov, M.D., is both an internist and a psychiatrist. Dr. Chertkov, do you have additional thoughts about the evaluation of this patient and treatment considerations?

Dr. Chertkov: Dr. Fleishman has done an excellent job of delineating a diagnostic framework and its use in patient assessment and in the development of a treatment plan. Such a framework is particularly vital in this setting in which a patient has multiple psychiatric symptoms in addition to chronic pain and a medical history that must be taken into account. This framework provides an opportunity to assess the patient's pain and the possible interplay of psychiatric and pain symptoms.

Importance of the Therapeutic Alliance

Successful treatment of chronic pain requires ongoing, effective communication; explicit discussion of the clinical process, emphasizing the crucial role of quality teamwork between the clinician and the patient in achieving treatment success; and clearly stated expectations about the process of assessing the efficacy of interventions. Management of chronic symptoms depends on collaborative work between the clinician and the patient, especially in the area of pain management, because communication of symptoms and side effects and evaluation of treatments require a strong therapeutic alliance. This patient, with a complex history of multiple losses and a real need to play an active role in her own care, must be encouraged to continue her current level of involvement in her own care and to work even more actively as her own advocate. Conveying respect for the vital role of the patient's self-evaluation and recording of the course of symptoms and treatment (e.g., through her pain diary) is especially important to ensure that the patient feels listened to and well cared for and to maximize the clinician's responsiveness to the patient's concerns. The addition of mood variables to the patient's pain diary, including scales of depression and anxiety, may help to identify the psychological distress caused by her pain symptoms, as well as the possible interplay of symptoms, and to provide opportunities for discussion of the psychological and interpersonal sequelae of chronic illness and the complexity of their interactions. It will also maximize the clinician's responsiveness to changes in symptoms or side effects and the clinician's ability to identify and address psychiatric symptoms.

Reinforce Successful Coping Strategies

The patient has described a pattern of recurrent pain episodes of extended duration with substantial associated functional limitation and poor response to pharmacological intervention. Exploration of her coping strategies may provide further helpful information about how she has tolerated these significant symptoms and may offer opportunities to reinforce existing coping skills, to explore potential avenues for further psychotherapeutic intervention, or to consider other treatment modalities. Given the patient's frustration with medications, and her strong self-motivation and self-discipline, she may be able to draw on her strengths and benefit from an exploration of alternative treatment modalities such as biofeedback and self-hypnosis, as well as relaxation therapies, acupuncture, or massage. Encouraging the patient to consider complementing her traditional therapies with other classes of interventions may support her sense of self-control and her active role in her own treatment and self-care. Complementary therapies do not substitute for the patient's aggressive pursuit of biomedical treatment but may support her existing tendency to consider all avenues of intervention, her long-standing coping skills, and her need for a variety of supportive treatments.

Other Diagnostic Considerations

Although the patient is frustrated by both her previous treatments and her diagnostic evaluations, the etiology of her pain syndrome remains unclear. Obviously, the primary, and most worrisome, concern is that her pain might reflect a recurrence of breast cancer or some new, and equally dangerous, underlying cause. Because her episodes of pain have varied in their quality, duration, and intensity, further diagnostic evaluation is necessary. The patient's presumptive diagnosis of herpes zoster as the cause of her pain may well be appropriate, but no confirmatory evidence for this diagnosis has been found, whether her pain symptoms have been dermatomal is not clear, and no herpetic lesions were seen at any time. As Dr. Fleishman has suggested, immediate review of the status of her breast disease is imperative, including review of appropriate scans. Although it may be anxiety-provoking to introduce the need for ongoing diagnostic evaluation as her symptoms evolve, recurrence of pain symptoms with so many differences in their characteristics necessitates further evaluation.

The patient's prior diagnosis of postherpetic neuralgia can prompt a certain complacency around her workup. In addition, we are well aware that pain syndromes in women have been traditionally underdiagnosed and underevaluated. Although an atypical presentation of cardiac disease and angina, gastroesophageal reflux disease, and a second cancer are far less likely etiologies of her distress based on her description of the pain symptoms, they should be entertained and ruled out. Osteoporosis and arthritis are far more common explanations of pain syndromes in elderly women, but even these conditions apparently have not been fully evaluated. Consultation with her internist should confirm results of her most recent mammogram, as well as other imaging studies that may need to be repeated. A comprehensive neurological examination should be performed in the setting of this recurrence of pain symptoms if one has not been done in recent months.

Talk of Suicide: Axis I or Axis II Disorder?

The patient's report of severe depressive symptoms and chronic suicidal ideation is particularly disturbing and quite anxiety-provoking for the consultant. Parallel history confirming patterns of suicidal or parasuicidal activity is imperative. The patient alluded to quite serious suicidal behavior that merited intensive care and for which she had presumed lethality. Interestingly, Dr. Fleishman confines his discussion of the patient's suicidality to his review of the management of Axis II concerns. However, her psychiatric history is insufficient to rule out the possibility that her suicide attempt occurred in the setting of a major depressive episode or in the presence of psychotic symptoms (less likely); we have not ruled out other risk factors for completed suicide (such as substance abuse or alcoholism); and whether the patient's condition meets criteria for an Axis I depressive disorder at this time is unclear. Further review of her psychiatric symptoms, along with an ongoing medical evaluation, is vital. Although major depression may be comorbid, and not a causal factor in her pain syndrome, its identification would dictate use of an antidepressant in the first phase of treatment, in addition to consideration of an anticonvulsant for analgesia. Assessment of depressive and psychotic symptoms, and other suicide risk factors, is essential to make a reasonable safety determination and disposition.

Although Dr. Fleishman assigned the patient a functional score of 85–90, she has described being bedridden during severe pain episodes, and her symptoms clearly cause her profound psychological distress. The timing and intensity of her evaluation and trials of treatments should be in keeping with the severity of her concerns. Chronic symptoms call for both patience and a sense of urgency—the acknowledgment that this has been a long-standing problem that has not responded adequately to first-line treatments requires a detailed, analytic approach but one that must take into account the patient's natural impatience with yet another long and protracted course. Delineating a long-term therapeutic plan, acknowledging the patient's frustration with previous treatments, and noting the likelihood that it may take time and substantial effort to achieve an adequate therapeutic outcome is essential. In a patient who is explicitly threatening suicide, reviewing anticipated potential problems and strategies for handling them and ensuring good communication are very important. One may hope for smooth sailing, but the management of long-standing chronic pain symptoms can be complex and wrought with conflicts. Assuring improvements in the patient's social support structure is an additional step that may contribute to her therapeutic goals.

The attribution of a personality disorder in th[
lematic. She may have some narcissistic feature[
comments and the elements of her history has[
ternative explanation. The patient is clearly a pr[
dent woman who has had a difficult life. Like m[
chronic pain, she has become frustrated with h[
mistic about interventions and the potential for improvement in
the future. Wishing to play an active role in treatment, to avoid
the unnecessary repetition of diagnostic tests and failed clinical
trials, and to avoid further psychotherapy or exploratory work do
not, in and of themselves, describe narcissism. Conflicts around
issues of dependency and control are classic in patients with
chronic pain symptoms, and her strong personality may, in fact,
have carried her through each of her multiple losses, and she can
be assured that it serves her well in this current challenge.

Case 2: Headaches in a Woman Who Arrives With a Provocative Introduction

Before starting your office hours on a Monday morning, you glance at the mail that you received over the weekend. Your eye catches a return address: B. B. William, Esq., Attorney-at-Law. The letter inside reads as follows:

Dear Doctor:

I am grateful that you will be seeing my sister, Mrs. Pilig, in consultation. I have encouraged her to seek psychiatric assistance for some time. As you will hear and see, she has many problems. I am quite sure that she will honestly describe her many previous surgeries and her current work pressures; she likely will accurately describe her migraine headaches which recently have become incapacitating. I am less confident that she will tell you about her history of drug abuse.

While in college and early during her marriage (now divorced), my sister began obtaining prescriptions from many doctors to treat her migraine headaches. She became addicted to barbiturates and several pain drugs. When she was in college, her friend summoned me to her home after she had been unable to reach my sister on the telephone for several days. I had to remove the bathroom door to find my sister incoherent, surrounded by pills and scratching her wrists with a razor blade. I took her for medical attention, but unfortunately the emergency om doctors did not admit her. She saw a psychiatrist only briefly at that time. I suspect that she had used drugs periodically for many years. Recently, I became distressed when I spoke with her on the phone at 10:00 A.M. on a Saturday morning and noticed that she had slurred speech and was talking in the nonsense way she used to talk when she was using drugs.

I hope this will be helpful; I do not mean to intrude into the doctor-patient relationship. However, if I can be of any assistance, please call me at 123-4567.

Sincerely yours,
B. B. William, Esq.
Attorney-at-Law

You note that your first patient is indeed the attorney's sister. Mrs. Pilig is an anorectic-appearing, tastefully and professionally dressed 48-year-old woman who describes her history in a disorganized, but friendly, way. She states that her gynecologist referred her to you when he learned that her migraine headaches had increased in frequency and intensity over the past year. She first developed incapacitating headaches in her mid-teens. She recalls having to spend 2–3 days in bed in a darkened room, often missing as many as 5 days of school because of a headache. Her headaches kept her from achieving success as a ballet dancer and as a student. She reports that she hated staying at home with her migraines because her alcoholic mother was "drunk much of the time," and the patient was expected to baby-sit her younger sister after school if she were home with a migraine. Mrs. Pilig attended a university away from home but left school after 5 years without a degree. She recalls that her headaches were always worse around examination time, and she relates her difficulty studying and completing her undergraduate degree to headaches.

In her mid-20s, Mrs. Pilig married a helicopter pilot. She describes her ex-husband with respect and kindness but is vague about why this marriage ended after 6 years. She recalls that her frequently incapacitating headaches persisted throughout her marriage. She also developed chronic indigestion and was given the diagnosis of gastric ulcers, ultimately requiring a vagotomy and then, later, a pyloroplasty in her early 30s. Since these surgeries, she has developed lactose intolerance and an inability to eat more than "a few mouthfuls" of food at one sitting. In her early 40s, she had a vaginal hysterectomy (ovaries left intact) for fibroids, and at age 46, she had a cholecystectomy for "gallstones." Mrs. Pilig sees her dermatologist regularly and has had "many little melanomas" removed from sun-exposed parts of her body.

When asked whether she has ever taken medications that helped with migraines or whether she has had any previous psychiatric contact, Mrs. Pilig states that she had seen a psychiatrist while in college for "about a session" but does not recall much about this treatment. She states that she received previous treatment with a number of medications but cannot name most of them. She does recall having taken Fiorinal and Valium, which seemed to help some with headaches. Recently, she has been attempting to treat her headaches with over-the-counter preparations (Motrin and Tylenol-PM). She states that she drinks alcohol rarely: "just a half a glass of wine at Christmas." Her description of her headaches is the classic description of migraines.

During the interview, Mrs. Pilig is smiling and cooperative but vague about her failed marriage and other relationships. She becomes quite animated when you inquire about her work. She is the office administrator for a political figure and has a 15-year history of dedicated service to her boss, whom she respects and cherishes. She admires his commitment to his work and his success. She has a "dreamy" look when she describes, at some length, his ability to combine attention to the pressures of political life with attention to his wife and children. She has missed very few days of work after her surgeries, and she misses only 1 workday a month because of her headaches. Because of her eating habits (described above), she is exhausted after work and on weekends. Mrs. Pilig states that she has few friends and interacts with her family "very little, because I really need my nights, weekends, and holidays to rest, so that I can get back to work." When asked if her weight is of concern to her, she smiles coyly and states that her brother, an attorney, has expressed concern that she may be malnourished. She also indicates that she is unable to climb one flight of stairs at work because the muscles in her legs are so weak.

On mental status examination, Mrs. Pilig appears neither depressed nor anxious. She checks her watch several times during the interview and reminds herself that she needs to get back to the office because her boss has an important meeting scheduled. She is fully oriented, has no obvious memory problems, and has no psychotic symptoms. She appears very fragile. As she schedules her next appointment with you, Mrs. Pilig states, "My brother will be very pleased that I came to see you; I told him I would tell you everything. Doctor, do you think medication could help my headaches?"

Dr. Massie: Philip R. Muskin, M.D., a psychoanalyst and consultation-liaison psychiatrist, discusses the evaluation and treatment of this patient, emphasizing countertransference reactions and potential treatment pitfalls.

Dr. Muskin: I have a visceral reaction to reading the letter; prior to knowing anything from the patient herself, I have a tight feeling in the pit of my stomach. I feel uncomfortable that I know things about this woman that she has not told me; how should I use information obtained outside of the interaction with the patient? The letter bears warnings that Mrs. Pilig will not be honest with me; that she has a history of addiction to several drugs, a strong indication of current drug use, and a history of at least one suicide attempt; and that she has not wanted psychiatric treatment. Communications such as this one may be an unsophisticated attempt to help the patient, but typically they indicate serious character problems in the author of the letter, in the identified patient, or in both parties. This warning comes from the patient's brother, the attorney. His intrusion into an evaluation and treatment that has not even started is unwanted and unsettling. Am I being put on notice? Will I be sued if I fail? What does failure mean, and who will make that determination? Is the brother telling me that this is a hopeless situation before I have even met the patient? The final reaction I have to the letter is one of sadness; I already have fantasies about this woman, even though we have never met. I wish that I had not read the letter; but I also hope that the patient will not keep her appointment.

However, the patient shows up and does live up to the fantasies. Her physical appearance suggests an eating disorder, and her history is both disorganized and lacking the information provided by her brother. My countertransference alarms go off because she appears as advertised. I realize that her gynecologist has not called me, suggesting that she may be hoping to stop seeing the patient, which is another bad sign.

Pain: An Idiom for Distress

Now I have a history from her, one that starts in the patient's teens and includes parental neglect and substance abuse, a suggestion of problematic interpersonal relationships, and failures secondary to her physical symptoms. How has pain become her primary symptom? As an idiom for distress, what does her pain describe? Does Mrs. Pilig have a history of physical or sexual abuse that she is not yet prepared to share or that she has repressed? I am impressed by her surgeries, at least five, and involving three or four organ systems. The description of her relationship with work and her employer, particularly her affect, seems idealized. Does work replace other relationships, and is intimacy preferable as a fantasy rather than in the reality of a true relationship with a person? My initial diagnostic impressions include a borderline personality disorder and a somatization disorder (Haase and Muskin, in press). She does not appear either depressed or anxious, which is a surprise, but I can be fooled in an initial consultation and reserve judgment until we have met more than once. How will Mrs. Pilig respond to my recommendations regarding her pain? Her response will give me a better idea of her mood than anything she presents in this initial visit. There is no surprise when she asks about medication for her headaches. However, I wonder what Mrs. Pilig has not told me because she claims that her pain does not interfere much with her life, and there seems little justification for her request for pain medication.

Forming a Therapeutic Alliance

The therapeutic approach to these types of patients is to attempt to form an alliance with them. I do not doubt that she is suffering, and I tell her so; however, I recommend that medication, particularly narcotic and/or sedative drugs, be used rarely in these circumstances. Mrs. Pilig has made a connection between increased pain and periods of increased stress in her life. Stress can be treated without pharmacological intervention because it is a psychological phenomenon. Is she amenable to talking about these situations as a way to help reduce her reaction to them? Adequate nutrition has been a problem, resulting in fatigue that she finds troublesome. Perhaps some help from a nutritionist (whom I know and have worked with before) would be of benefit. I also need more information about Mrs. Pilig's previous treatments. Has she ever been given medications for her pain, and have there been any problems with or resulting from the medications? This offers an opportunity for her to tell me about her prior addictions, or not. It is important that Mrs. Pilig understand that I see her as someone who struggles with pain, a struggle that takes courage. There is no issue regarding the "reality" of the pain—her pain is real, period. This must be made crystal clear to her, or no therapy is possible.

Discussing Information Obtained From a Third Party

Mrs. Pilig does not appear to have many relationships with other people outside of her idealized relationship at work. Her marriage failed. What role did she play in that? At this stage, I would bring up the letter from her brother; does she know that he had written to me? What does Mrs. Pilig think her brother felt was important that I know about her? Because the letter suggests far greater incapacity than Mrs. Pilig has described, and also indicates possible current substance abuse, it cannot remain a secret. To do so would destroy any trust this patient might develop in me. In my head echoes, "And what a wicked web we weave, when first we try to deceive." If I am deceptive with her, I should expect the same in return. Her response to the letter may be the strongest predictor of the outcome of the treatment. Anger would be the best reaction but should be tempered with the realization that her brother must be concerned about her. If she denies everything in the letter, that is fine. Sadness that her brother did not trust her but that what he said is accurate would be ideal, and ideal is another word for fantasy. Patients change their story many times in therapy as they understand themselves and their motivations, as they are able to face what has happened in their lives, and as they trust the therapist enough to stop censoring. Given her history of self-harm and substance use, I would confront her denial of current substance use with her brother's impression that she was intoxicated recently. If she lies to me, the likelihood of success is much reduced, but it is not zero because we have just begun to work together. The most negative predictive sign would be a manipulative and seductive response to the letter.

Self-Hypnosis: A Technique to Gain Control

My final recommendation for this initial consultation is that Mrs. Pilig be taught hypnosis as a way to control her pain. Hypnosis offers patients a method to take control over their pain without the side effects, potential addiction, and limitations of medications. Pain is experienced as something that controls the individual; hypnosis offers a way to wrest control back. I would teach hypnosis in the same way that I would prescribe a medication for her; it is part of the therapy. I hope to communicate with the intact part of her ego; her response will provide some indication of whether I have succeeded.

At this point, Mrs. Pilig's psychodynamics are unclear. There are suggestions and vague impressions but nothing to aid in creating the psychological story of her life. I plan to learn this story over the next several sessions, assuming she agrees to this approach. Mrs. Pilig's unwillingness to participate in treatment after her suicide attempt may or may not predict how she will experience psychotherapy at this point in her life. The symptoms she communicates and presents as I get to know her will determine the necessary pharmacological intervention. If she has significant mood symptoms, I will recommend an antidepressant, but which one will be dictated by her concerns about side effects, particularly sexual side effects and weight gain. Does her being slender mean she wishes to look this way, or is her appearance ego-dystonic? If Mrs. Pilig has significant mood lability, a mood stabilizer would be a consideration. If she insists on narcotic or sedative medication and will accept no other therapy, then this becomes the most difficult situation. If Mrs. Pilig wants stronger pain medications, given that she has told me that she has been managing without these classes of medications, then I am not the right therapist for her. If she is willing to give up the opportunity to be better, not necessarily pain-free (I try never to promise something that is impossible to deliver) and not bound to drugs that ultimately will cause her more problems, I cannot help her. If Mrs. Pilig is willing to try, I believe that her pain can be reduced and that she can control it rather than having it control her. The choice is not mine; it is hers.

Dr. Massie: Dr. Chertkov has additional management suggestions for this complex patient.

Dr. Chertkov: Dr. Muskin masterfully describes the range of possible countertransference reactions evoked by this patient and her initial presentation, preceded by a letter of warning from her attorney brother. Dr. Muskin's illustration of these strong emotions, and his description of his own analytic process of exploring his countertransference, provides a framework to understand the issues raised in treating this complex patient. Mrs. Pilig's history raises several complex concerns because it includes chronic pain symptoms; a pattern of help-seeking; medical intervention, including multiple surgeries; substance abuse; resistance to psychiatric treatment; an eating disorder; the question of a trauma history; the negotiation of complex family relationships; establishment of a therapeutic alliance in the setting of conflicting history; and confidentiality concerns. In fact, the array of problems and the complexity of the countertransference described may leave one feeling overwhelmed, already hopeless and frustrated about the potential for treatment success, and resentful of the referring physician who has chosen to remain uninvolved even in the referral process itself.

Perhaps most striking in considering this case is the absolute necessity of establishing a clinical framework as a basis for exploring and understanding the large amount of information already available about this patient. Such a framework allows one to be acutely aware of transference issues, while attending to the need for ongoing, self-critical analysis of the ways in which these feelings may already be shaping the therapeutic interaction. The feelings of anxiety and anger that Dr. Muskin explores offer clues to possible pitfalls in this patient's future care and identify factors that may have contributed to past treatment failures.

Drug Abuse or Inadequate Pain Relief?

The need for further history is paramount. It is unclear whether this patient's primary problem is substance abuse or whether this patient, in the setting of chronic pain, has been inappropriately accused of abusing drugs or being dependent on them because of behaviors that are common because of inadequate pain relief.

Thus, patients whose pain has not been appropriately managed may appear to be abusing drugs as they demand more medications, become anxious about the availability of refills, stockpile against the eventuality of a dreaded pain crisis, and self-dose more frequently or at higher levels than are prescribed because of poor symptom control. This so-called medication-seeking behavior may have manipulative features, evoking anger among clinicians and resentment about dependency issues. However, physiological dependence on appropriate analgesia is a normal feature of long-term use of opiates and other pain medications and, as has been well described in earlier chapters, does not indicate a substance abuse problem and is not a contraindication to aggressive treatment. Collecting a clear medical history, including parallel history from family and previous clinicians, will help to clarify this patient's management.

Obtain a More Detailed History

Dr. Muskin's case discussion has focused on countertransference, and a great deal of detailed information has already been presented; however, the history has fundamental gaps, and we need a complete mental status examination, review of systems (both medical and psychiatric), discussion of current medications (including traditional and alternative therapies), and identification of current and previous medical caregivers.

The medical management of this patient's pain syndrome is unclear. Although her primary complaint is headaches, whether the headaches are migraine type or whether she has had adequate trials of migraine prophylaxis (e.g., β–blockers) is unknown. All treatment with pain medications, including dosages and duration, must be clarified. The patient's previous medical records may help to detail her pain history because she cannot recall many of the specifics of a more than 20-year course of symptoms and treatments. Her medical care and surgeries are impressive, but many of her symptoms have a disturbingly common theme in that they are highly associated with anxiety disorders and depression; and, by her own report, she has never had adequate psychiatric care. Research about abdominal and pelvic pain in women, and the connections between psychiatric and gastrointestinal symptoms, is ongoing, but many questions remain unanswered. Mrs. Pilig's journey, including multiple surgical procedures, is not an uncommon one. Unfortunately, the limits of medical knowledge, biases about substance abuse, and tendency to label women as hysterical in their presentation of symptoms have contributed to long-standing failure to correctly diagnose pain syndromes in women (e.g., anginal syndromes), inappropriate gynecological surgeries, and undertreatment of chronic pain.

An Opportunity to Explore Family Conflicts and Concern

The letter from the patient's brother presents an intriguing problem, providing potentially critical information about her history, including substance abuse and self-injurious or suicidal behavior, and placing the clinician in a difficult position of negotiating complex family dynamics in the setting of an initial encounter. Dr. Muskin correctly asserts that avoiding deception is essential to establishing a therapeutic alliance that will form the basis of a successful treatment. Openly sharing the letter with the patient, acknowledging the emotional challenges attendant with doing so, and inviting her comments will provide a wealth of information. The assurance that her discussions with you are confidential will allow the explicit delineation of a therapeutic frame, encourage her to trust the bounds of her relationship with you, enable her to identify that she is the primary patient, and clarify that you will consider her brother's letter within the context of her relationship with you and that you value her assessment of its contents. This may provide an opportunity for Mrs. Pilig to begin to share elements of her history that she did not initially disclose. Alternatively, she may offer a different interpretation of those events or may deny that they occurred, providing you with a valuable perspective on family conflicts. With her permission, you may want to consider a range of quite different options, including planning a family session, informing the brother that your contacts with Mrs. Pilig are confidential and that you appreciate his concern but cannot have further interactions with him without her explicit permission, or encouraging her to work with you on addressing her brother's concerns. While interactions with lawyers, either as patients or family members, may evoke anxiety in the treating clinician, it is important to critically assess these feelings, carefully identifying the countertransference themes and obtaining assistance with or supervision around them if they become problematic. The family or individual disturbance reflected in this correspondence is difficult to assess, and there is a very real danger that the fears elicited in the therapist may inappropriately color the interpretation of events.

The "Ideal" Therapist for the Patient With Pain

Dr. Muskin concludes with the suggestion that he can endeavor to assist this patient, but the core choices are hers. His suggestion that "if Mrs. Pilig wants stronger pain medications,…then I am not the right therapist for her" is problematic because we do not yet have a clear history of the pharmacological interventions that have been tried or a sense of the full range of treatment that she may require to obtain pain relief. Clinicians' level of comfort with a range of pain therapies varies; however, regardless of the severity of this patient's symptoms, or the possible range of etiologies or treatments, Dr. Muskin probably is, in fact, the ideal therapist for her. His strong concern about a range of complex aspects of Mrs. Pilig's care is evident in his case discussion, and his awareness and clear presentation of these countertransference issues offer the best chance to use them effectively in the treatment and to achieve therapeutic success.

Case 3: Fibromyalgia in a "Super-Responsible" Woman With a History of Treatment by Multiple Physicians

Your new patient, a moderately obese, smiling 42-year-old junior high school administrator dressed in colorful, casual attire presents to her first session accompanied by her courteous husband. She states with a twinkle in her eye, "my life is a total mess, but isn't everyone's?" The patient relates that she was referred by her breast surgeon. She had been seeing another psychiatrist intermittently but feels that it is "time for a change." Her last psychiatrist had helped her adjust to "disastrous plastic surgery results" after a bilateral prophylactic mastectomy that she had chosen to have to reduce her risk of dying from breast cancer as had her mother. The patient states that the breast reconstruction went very badly; she had the implants removed, and she will likely be unable to have further breast reconstruction. She smilingly describes a "totally frustrating 2 years of depositions" prior to her "dropping" her lawsuit against her plastic surgeon.

The patient states that she was referred to you "to see if I'm on the right medications for fibromyalgia." Her previous psychiatrist had prescribed amitriptyline (175 mg at night) as a hypnotic, alprazolam (1 mg four times a day), and paroxetine (40 mg/day). She regulates her dose of amitriptyline and alprazolam "depending on the day" and cannot remember yesterday's dose. In addition, she takes methocarbamol for pain, which was prescribed by her neurologist who "never felt it was important" for him to speak with her many other doctors. The patient states that her fibromyalgia was diagnosed by a neurologist whom she consulted for evaluation of acute neck pain resulting from a work injury. She indicates that her injury clearly resulted from negligence in the workplace; however, she "didn't have the energy to sue."

The patient states, "I've got a lot of pain, but the fibromyalgia is the worst." She recalls having developed migraine headaches as a teenager, and these incapacitating migraines continue to occur about monthly. She has "sciatic pain that comes and goes" and is described as "totally, totally horrible right now." She has had "several" epidural analgesia injections over the past 3 months for "a bad disk, but I won't have surgery." Her symptoms of fibromyalgia include chronic fatigue, multiple tender points (she gestures to her shoulders, neck, lumbar spine, and hips), "arthritic joint pain," and disrupted sleep (which she describes as much improved with amitriptyline). "My psychiatrist had me up to 200 mg once, but I was too zonked during the day." She misses approximately 4 workdays a month because of her pain and uses her summer months of school vacation as a time to "sleep and do absolutely nothing." She states that she is never really free from pain. She has seen "more neurologists than I can count" for her 25-year history of pain and describes dissatisfaction with most. In the past, she has been prescribed lorazepam, cyclobenzaprine, oxycodone and acetaminophen, oxycodone and aspirin, belladonna, and "a lot of other stuff." She takes estrogen and progesterone for menopausal symptoms that developed at age 36. She states that her current neurologist is not encouraging about her consideration of continued psychiatric assistance. She states, "I'm not depressed, and that's not what the paroxetine is for; it does something chemically for fibromyalgia." In addition, the patient sees at least two, maybe three, internists for her general health care. One has diagnosed "borderline kidney function" and has advised that she never take acetaminophen-containing drugs.

The patient's descriptions of her various pain syndromes are vague; she has difficulty remembering names of doctors, diagnostic tests, past procedures to treat pain, and medications. She corrects herself multiple times as she describes the effects of medications and their side effects, and she is vague about the success or failure of previous trigger point injections, spinal analgesia, acupuncture, and chiropractic spine manipulations. She seems suggestible, and, at times, she appears to be guessing at and providing the response she believes you would want to hear.

Both of the patient's parents are deceased, and she has no siblings. She has been married for 20 years to a man she describes as "brilliant and the most wonderful father"; however, later in the interview, she expresses dissatisfaction with her marriage, his career and current financial situation, and his lack of participation in household chores and responsibility for planning of social activities. She is extremely proud of her only child, a teenage son. None of her immediate family members has any pain syndrome. She and her husband have been the "super-responsible" relatives who have felt obligated to provide both financial and practical assistance to aging aunts and uncles. "He gives them the money we really don't have to give away, and I, of course, do all of the work." She hates her job but loves working with children. "I can't stop working now; frankly, we need my salary." Over the past 3 years, she has given up a busy social schedule of friendship and church activities because "I'm so exhausted all the time." Initially, she described her husband's and her own lack of association with others as resulting from their decision to "reevaluate and reprioritize our lives." However, later in the interview, she describes their lack of socialization as related to her husband's depressed mood, which has been apparent to her for the last several years.

The patient appears neither depressed nor anxious. She is "smilingly sarcastic" as she describes her history. At times, it is difficult for you to know if she is using humor, imprecise language, or sarcasm. As you attempt to clarify her statements, she becomes apologetic ("I'm making this so hard for you, aren't I?") and then recants. She is fully oriented, and no past or current psychotic symptoms are evident. At the end of the session, she eagerly schedules the next appointment but indicates that she will have to call to confirm because she forgot her appointment book. The patient also indicates that she forgot to check whether she is running out of her medications, but she believes that she will need to call you and ask you to refill these prescriptions. She states that from the little time she has spent with you that she already sees that you are "exactly the person I am looking for, and I came here with great confidence in you because you are so highly recommended." Her final question is, "Doctor, do you think that you can help me with this pain?"

Dr. Massie: Randy S. Roth, Ph.D., an expert in fibromyalgia and other pain disorders, describes a comprehensive approach to "pain control" in this patient with hysteroid personality features.

Dr. Roth: This patient, who presents with a chief complaint of fibromyalgia embedded in a larger context of multiple somatic complaints, a conviction of severe physiological breakdown, apparent cooperation with numerous physicians and treatment regimens without symptomatic improvement, and multilevel psychological disturbance, represents a difficult and challenging case. In comparison with most cases of fibromyalgia, this case is atypical because of the obvious lack of affective distress (depression is an expected secondary clinical sign in fibromyalgia). Most clinicians are familiar with the daunting challenge of bringing to health a patient who reports serious somatic concerns but who, nonetheless, appears to have little of the affective distress that is typically associated with their illness. It is not surprising that clinicians become suspicious about the motivation of such a patient to seek improved health and function, and an inference of significant psychopathology with a corollary skepticism regarding the validity of the patient's complaints is often, and appropriately, made. Moreover, this patient has character features that further place her readiness for meaningful treatment into question, such as her gratuitous interactional style with the interviewer; her tendency toward idealization of significant others (e.g., her husband, the interviewer); her colorful, diffuse, and extreme descriptions of her history of victimization (e.g., "disastrous plastic surgery," "totally frustrating 2 years of depositions," "my life is a total mess," "totally, totally horrible" sciatica); and her denial of psychological problems. More commonly, patients with fibromyalgia present with obvious depression and distress, without the hysteroid personality features so apparent in this woman. As a result, psychiatric intervention must target these personality characteristics, as well as her pain, to achieve a successful outcome.

Clinical Features and Diagnostic Considerations

However, several clinical features in this patient are prevalent among women with fibromyalgia, who constitute 90% of the population of fibromyalgia patients. These women often have a long history of sacrifice and an overdeveloped sense of duty and responsibility, to the detriment of their physical and psychological health. Often, they are working mothers who are single or who have an uninvolved spouse. Life demands are great or overwhelming, time constraints are constant and compelling, and an extended pattern of inadequate sleep coupled with rare opportunities for rest and leisure from work and family obligations is common. This pattern leads to impaired stress tolerance and mood functioning. Developmentally, it is not uncommon to observe a childhood history noteworthy for untoward responsibility at an early age, inadequate parental nurturance, excessive overt or covert parental criticism, and/or frank abuse. This emotional environment often is further complicated by a biological history prevalent for major affective disorder. Taken together, these individuals as adults have an extraordinary need to please others, are subassertive, harbor a devalued self-worth, and are obsessive and intropunitive while maintaining a posture of social desirability and convention. However, a martyrdom-like demeanor and a submerged bitterness can be observed by the astute clinician. Self-reward and self-nurturance are "totally" sacrificed for the good of others. These clinical signs are illustrated in this present case by the patient's self-description of being "super-responsible," her obligatory caretaking of extended family members, the need to use her somatic symptoms to justify a summer vacation of leisure and rest, and her failure to assertively address her perception of nonsupport from her husband. These observations are not pathognomonic of fibromyalgia, but they are all too common among those patients who seek treatment.

Her diffuse pain complaints of myalgias and arthralgias and the presence of tender points appear to meet the criteria for fibromyalgia. She has a history of migraine headache, which is frequently a comorbid symptom of fibromyalgia. Whether she actually has sciatica is unclear, although her symptoms were sufficiently impressive to convince a pain specialist to administer "spinal analgesia" (probably an epidural steroid nerve block). Of note, the original diagnosis of fibromyalgia was made by a neurologist during evaluation of an acute cervical injury. Whether the diagnosis of fibromyalgia was based on a soft-tissue neck injury or her more diffuse complaints of pain is not stated in the case description. Regional, nonneurological, musculoskeletal pain is commonly misdiagnosed as fibromyalgia when the problem is actually myofascial pain. Her history of injection of trigger points (which give rise to referred pain) compared with the presence of tender points (which do not) further suggests a myofascial component to her pain. In this regard, a piriformis myofascial syndrome would mimic the lower-extremity pain often mistaken for lumbar radiculopathy and might account for her "sciatica."

Pharmacologic Treatment

In considering treatment of these symptoms, modification of her pharmacological regimen is not likely to significantly reduce her pain or attendant disability. An alternative TCA or another antidepressant, singly or in combination, may be more efficacious; her current regimen is optimal based on current empirical studies. TCAs, in general, and amitriptyline, more specifically, have been the most exhaustively studied of the psychotropic agents for the treatment of fibromyalgia and are by far the most clinically significant in controlled trials (Max 1995). The efficacy of selective serotonin reuptake inhibitors alone for the treatment of fibromyalgia is as yet not well supported by empirical study, although the addition of a selective serotonin reuptake inhibitor to a TCA may have additive clinical benefits (Goldenberg et al. 1996). Alprazolam has been found helpful in one fibromyalgia study, but minor tranquilizers in fibromyalgia have not been systematically investigated. It is noteworthy that this patient takes methocarbamol "for pain," a muscle relaxant that is contraindicated for chronic use. In my experience, dependence on muscle relaxants for chronic musculoskeletal pain likely reflects central tranquilizing effects under the guise of medical therapy and portends poor treatment outcome. Given the significant psychological issues inherent in this patient's clinical presentation, I am skeptical that a strictly medical solution will promote a dramatic change in her symptoms.

Establishing Rapport and Strategic Therapy

From a psychotherapeutic standpoint, the most crucial (and most difficult) objective is to establish a productive therapeutic alliance that has the potential for behavior change. The patient's long history of medical treatment without symptomatic improvement is striking. Any early suggestion of a psychological contribution to her pain is likely to be met with resistance and thwart further therapeutic efforts. In fact, one might surmise that, despite her apparent request for help in pain control, her chief, albeit unconscious, clinical motive is to remain in treatment and maintain her pain. Her idealized impression of the interviewer as "exactly the person I am looking for" is a clear warning for the subsequent passive sabotage of therapy. These patients present perplexing obstacles for the clinician who can be easily seduced by such gratuitous remarks.

In such cases, I find the strategic therapy approach (Fisch et al. 1982) to be very helpful in treating covert resistance and facilitating clinical gains without explicitly addressing psychological dysfunctions that are ego-dystonic for the patient. This therapeutic model emphasizes the use of concrete behavioral assignments, speaking in the patient's "language" (thus, the early focus on salient behavioral attributes offered by the patient), and paradoxical directive, in addition to the use of metaphoric language in promoting behavior change. I would, thus, adopt a "one-down" position with this patient that discourages overly optimistic expectations about treatment or my ability to help. If her symptoms are viewed as a tactic of control in the therapeutic relationship, whereby maintenance of her symptoms permits her to retain control over the therapeutic agenda, overt and overly aggressive maneuvers to reduce her symptoms might jeopardize her control and enhance her resistance. In other words, expectations that her symptoms must be relinquished might disarm her. By avoiding this potential pitfall, treatment can proceed without overt challenge to her "right" to maintain her symptoms. Thus, I would carefully avoid making "pain relief" a stated goal of therapy but rather "pain control." In the early sessions, I would emphasize those aspects of the patient's self-view that are most salient (e.g., ego-syntonic), such as her commitment to "super-responsibility," her vocational and parental accomplishments, and her courage to seek mastectomy for her long-term health needs. By accepting these psychological attributes, but noting how extreme they can become, the stage is set for modestly modifying them to fall within more "healthy" limits, without identifying them as pathological. In addition, I would educate her about the nature of fibromyalgia as a disorder of pain modulation often occurring in women who have "taken on the burdens" but at the cost of "burnout of the nervous system." In essence, she is "out of balance" both somatically and emotionally. Thus, "rebalancing" her lifestyle is the prescription for "recalibrating the nervous system." These metaphors can serve as the justification and framework for interventions to follow that target psychological and physiological restoration. This also shifts the psychiatric perspective away from personality aberrations or mood disturbances that are likely to be perceived as too threatening.

Further Therapeutic Considerations

Pain treatment interventions that can be framed within this "restoration" paradigm, and that are standard for chronic pain management, include relaxation training, cognitive-behavioral strategies to "increase pain tolerance" (such as distraction, reducing catastrophizing, enhancing perceived control), therapeutic exercise (including both stretching and aerobics for myofascial and

fibromyalgia pain, which may require a referral to either a physical therapist or a physiatrist), and increasing participation in leisure activities. Slowly and gradually, by committing the patient
to specific tasks associated with alterations in behavior based
around the concept of "restoration of the nervous system," it is
hoped that a trusting therapeutic alliance can be established and
significant behavioral changes will occur to reduce both physical
and psychological morbidity.

At the appropriate time, the marital discord must be addressed.
Perhaps the patient will voluntarily bring it up, or it may come
up during an unrelated discussion. The marital relationship is
likely a perpetuating factor in maintaining the patient's symptoms. Her illness complaints may, in part, represent her reactions
to her husband's depression and his withdrawal of attention and
affection. Treatment of his depression through individual psychiatric care and/or marital therapy may be critical to ensure maintenance of any obtained therapeutic gains for both partners.

Conclusion

The therapist needs to walk the tightrope between the obvious
nature of the patient's psychological dysfunction and her avoidance of it. Sober treatment goals, patience, and a realistic appraisal
of the very difficult challenges that come with managing such
chronic-pain patients are necessary attitudes to sustain the clinician willing to practice in the "pain game."

Case 4: A Man With Back Pain:
A Family "Buys In"

You are asked by your colleague, an internist with whom you
share office space, to see a patient on whom he has just consulted.
The busy internist states, "I'm glad you can see him this morning. I am not sure that his wife will be able to get him back to
you. He is a 45-year-old schoolteacher who has lived with chronic low back pain, if you call it living, for 20-odd years. His wife
brought him here because of his right ankle pain. I just diagnosed
gout, drew bloods, and prescribed allopurinol. While in the
army 20 years ago, he was in an automobile accident that result-

ed in a fractured hip; his right leg is an inch shorter than his left. He has a family history of depression and appears to be quite depressed. This kind of patient scares me; I wonder if he just might kill himself."

You interview the patient and his wife together at the patient's insistence. The patient is uncomfortable talking about his pain, his family history, and himself. The history you are able to obtain is as follows: this married father of two children has a master's degree and is a dedicated, overly responsible, reliable junior high school teacher. His chronic back pain limits all activities; it forces him to go to bed to read and rest as soon as he comes home from teaching, and he remains in bed much of the time on the weekend. He and his wife have no friends and have had virtually no social contacts for the last 5–8 years. The family has been unable to take a vacation for many years because of his chronic back pain and flare-ups of gout that seem to occur before any planned vacation or any holiday. Because of his chronic back pain, he engages in no athletic, religious, or volunteer activities. When you comment that it seems he has "given up much in life," his prim wife rapidly responds, "fortunately, we are people with few wants. We have two lovely children, and they are excellent students, straight A students. The children and I pitch in to take care of the home and the yard." When you ask the patient why he had not presented for evaluation of these problems earlier, the wife quickly answers, "my husband was treated with so many pain medications in the hospital at the time he was injured that he is allergic to virtually all medications; they all give him an upset stomach." The patient nods authoritatively to this response.

The patient reluctantly describes his family history. He was born in the Midwest. His father died at age 45 of a myocardial infarction after years of incapacitating cardiac symptoms. The patient's mother and sister have both attempted suicide by overdose. Apparently, they were treated with antidepressant medication. However, this couple is very vague about their symptoms and treatments because "some family things are just best not to meddle in." Although the patient prefers to describe his distress in terms of his physical discomfort, he has at least a 25-year history of recurrent depressive disorder that has been undiagnosed and untreated. He has had months of "down moods," insomnia, early-morning awakening, decreased concentration, and irritability. Because of his back pain, he has been unable to accept promotions at work that would have provided additional money for the family. He sees this as a "failure," and he imagines that, in some ways, his family would be "better off without him." He has no clear history of suicide attempts or a current plan for suicide. Although he and his wife describe their lack of socialization with friends and family as related to his chronic back pain and need for bed rest, the patient's wife hints about episodes of severe anxiety that develop if they attempt to walk even a few blocks to a function at the home of a colleague. The wife indicates that the patient "clutches his chest" and that they must "run home as fast as they can" so the patient "can calm down and get control of himself." The patient casts a disapproving glance at his wife as she makes these remarks.

The patient appears tense, aloof, and somewhat irritable. He is wearing a business suit, and he sits and stands erectly. When his wife is speaking, he rocks back and forth in his chair and slaps his thigh with his hand. His speech is precise, articulate, and goal-directed, and no psychotic thought process or content is evident. He appears depressed and has a constricted range of affect. He is neither uncooperative nor forthcoming. His wife appears eager to provide added details; however, she frequently glances at her husband, searching for a clue from him about the appropriateness of her speaking. The couple shows no pleasantness or affection toward each other. Although he has been a chain-smoker for 30 years, the patient never drinks alcohol and takes no medication. He is easily 40–50 pounds overweight. His wife, a normal-weight woman, quips "we indulge little in life; at least we have good food on the table." The patient abruptly terminates the interview because he does not feel well. His wife seems surprised, but she rapidly collects their belongings and attempts to assist her husband in putting on his coat. The wife schedules a follow-up appointment with you in 1 week. She asks if she should attend the next session and, as they exit your office, asks "Doctor, do you think that there is something that could be done about his back pain?"

Dr. Massie: Barbara Kamholz, M.D., an expert in consultation psychiatry who incorporates family assessments into her treatment, provides an elegant summary of the approach to a family "suffering with pain."

Dr. Kamholz: This case appears to be a good example of "systems pathology," in which one individual is identified as having "the problem," but in reality the situation is better described as involving the entire family. This patient's "illness" is the dominating force in all of this family's daily activities and has been so for many years. Generally, long-term stable patterns of behavior that, on the surface, appear very dysfunctional in fact represent the satisfaction of complex, largely unconscious, needs. After many years, it can be very difficult to understand how the patterns originated and what needs they serve. The longevity and extent of the pattern—regardless of the etiology of the "pain"—make change difficult and indicate the need for a more rigorous and comprehensive, and probably long-term, therapeutic approach.

Discussion of the "Problem"

In approaching this situation, much care must be taken at the outset to avoid labeling the problem as exclusively "psychiatric" or "medical" because either approach will set the stage for therapeutic failure. This patient and his family have identified the patient's problems as physiological and likely will not readily accept the idea that the pain is "functional" or "psychiatric." However, trying to form an alliance with the family group by approaching the problem as a purely "medical" one at the outset may cause them to feel "betrayed" later when the functional issue of the effect of the patient's "pain" on the family is addressed (Roth and Kamholz 1997). Therefore, I would adopt an empathic, collaborative, nonthreatening stance, which labels the pain as a "significant problem" with "many effects" that will need to be "thoroughly investigated." Such an approach gives several strong signals to the family, including that the physician is very concerned about the suffering; that it is a serious issue that warrants careful attention and is *not* limited to the symptoms of "pain" (but not specified yet, either, so as not to encourage rejection of treatment by the family); and that there is hope for significant improvement "across the board," which will address many unconscious needs, thereby improving the therapeutic alliance. This first step is the most difficult and "tricky" one, and vague but meaningful comments are by far the most helpful at this stage. They allow the physician to refer the patient to an orthopedist and perhaps a neurologist *without* automatically ruling out a future psychiatric referral or solution.

I would certainly seek a referral to a physical medicine and rehabilitation specialist, and possibly a neurologist, as soon as possible. This patient has a history of an accident, differential leg lengths, and obesity; these factors suggest the potential for a myofascial pain syndrome with associated compensatory musculoskeletal abnormalities. Physical rehabilitation may offer him significant benefit. Furthermore, an immediate referral shows the family that the problem is being taken seriously; and, of course, the physician must know about any possible structural reasons for this man's back pain. As we know, chronic pain and depression are highly comorbid (Fisch et al. 1982), and although this family's problem might be readily interpreted as the result of "purely psychological" forces, an initiating, physiological event is often associated with real pain, which "sets the stage" for the development of broader-based family pathology.

The Pathology Extends Beyond the Patient

I would describe this family as pathologically organized because the needs of only one member are its primary focus. It appears that this patient dominates his family, not only by his helpless symptoms of pain and depression but also in the interpretation of reality. We observe this in the wife's careful checking with him for permission in speaking and in her protection of his world view. She accepts unquestioningly that his symptoms render him helpless, she readily accepts that his phobic anxiety (perhaps agoraphobia) about socializing is a "fact" of life, and she does not question his need to abruptly terminate the interview because he is not feeling well. She easily defends his solitary lifestyle and obesity by her quip, "we indulge little in life; at least we have good food on the table." That this view of a "reality defined by impairment" is shared is further observed in the unquestioning reaction of this couple's children. The children appear to have carefully designed their lives to minimize their needs and to prevent the addition of any further "problems" for the family; they are model children and assist with all the work at home. Notably, these behavior patterns—loyalty, service, unselfishness, and responsibility—are sufficiently socially synchronous that they would never be questioned except by a most perceptive family member, friend, or perhaps religious counselor. But in this context, they represent a severe distortion of family priorities and have seriously limited the choices available to the children.

But the Family "Buys Into It" Also

One of the perplexities of this all-too-common clinical situation is that family members do not "buy" into this system unless they too derive some benefit. This perspective allows us to understand that although the "patient" appears to be the primary benefactor, he is also a victim of his own pathology. It is clear that this system must in some way benefit all, and in fact the "patient" is trapped. It may not be immediately clear how this has developed, but a hypothesis could include the notions that such a structure has prevented the children from taking the risks of venturing outside the home, may have minimized parental conflicts or arguments, or may have prevented a dependent wife from having to develop her own life options, this equilibrium clearly will not be easily changed. Change will require each family member to question his or her own goals and needs and to have the courage and support to step forward and challenge the current family role definition. It is here that the therapist's main work will reside, and this need applies whether this patient's original problem was physiological *or* "functional" (Goldenberg et al. 1996; Max 1995).

A Diagnostic Formulation

A more traditional formulation of this patient's illness will of course include the potential for physiological causes of pain, but his psychological *reaction* to that pain also must be described. Classically speaking, the patient in this case is best described diagnostically on Axis I as having a pain disorder because his symptoms appear to meet the DSM-IV criteria: "pain in one or more anatomical sites" is a predominant focus of attention, the pain causes significant distress and impairment of function, psychological factors are clearly important in the maintenance of this problem, the symptom is not consciously derived, and the pain is not solely due to another Axis I disorder. However, this patient could also be fairly well described on Axis I as having a major depressive disorder, with prominent symptoms of insomnia, poor concentration, irritability, worthlessness, and hopelessness, with additional symptoms of anhedonia, social withdrawal, limited range of affect, and agoraphobia. In this regard, the family history of major depressive illness is most important. Of course, the diagnoses of pain disorder and depression are not mutually exclusive. Clearly, of these two disorders, his major depressive disorder offers more hope for immediate treatment pharmacologically.

A differential for Axis II diagnoses would include narcissistic personality disorder and obsessive-compulsive personality disorder, although many of these traits are shared by patients with depression, and they may be mutable with treatment of the depression.

Other Aspects of the History

Other aspects of this patient's history are very worthy of exploration, particularly the family contexts in which his mother's and sister's suicidal ideation evolved. This patient may feel that depression is an expectation within his family, that it is a very comfortable "role" that has been rewarded. It is also intriguing that this patient's father died of a severe illness at precisely his own age. It is often very difficult for children to outlive their parents; they may feel disloyal and guilty as "survivors." This may be especially true in this case because this patient's chronic "physiological disability" may have occurred as "modeling" behavior associated with his father's chronic disability. This patient also may be angry with his father for "dying early" and may be "paying" for this anger psychologically by suffering the same fate at the same time that he is expressing "loyalty" by his emulation. In either case, these psychological factors can intensify the need to maintain current roles and relationships.

Finally, this family likely will reject referral to psychiatry outright because such a referral could be enormously threatening to their "self-definition." Thus, I believe the psychiatrist should counsel the internist to develop a treatment plan as follows.

Suggested Intervention Plan

1. *Initial approach by internist:* The physician should use empathic, supportive statements of concern that do not threaten the

family but express interest and a desire to help, and should refer the patient to a physical medicine and rehabilitation specialist and possibly a neurologist for workup of back pain, if this has not been done, with appropriate subsequent referrals. The physician most likely will need to provide some initial treatment of the pain, involving medication such as acetaminophen with codeine or nonsteroidal anti-inflammatory drugs. Amitriptyline and nortriptyline are also very good treatments for chronic pain, but any antidepressant may be rejected at this stage if the patient suspects that the physician thinks his symptoms are "not real, but just psychological." Therefore, the suggestion to use antidepressants, even if purely for pain, must be handled very carefully at this stage. The response of the family at this time will be important in determining how well they will tolerate an "investigation" into all of the issues relating to the pain. Paradoxically, they may well resist it as it will threaten their lifestyle. If internists detect such resistance, they may anticipate quite a "rough road" but must try to keep the family in treatment.

2. If the family *will* accept further evaluation of the "pain problem," the physician must determine whether they will settle for just treatment of the back pain or if they will also allow treatment of the patient's depression. Such a discussion could be initiated with comments such as "You know, when people have suffered for so long, the suffering itself can take on a life of its own. I have seen this many times, and it can often lead to depression. This is quite a normal response, but nonetheless we can offer treatment for it. There is no need for you to have this additional problem, and it can only make recovery all the more difficult." These comments clearly leave open the (later) possibility of identifying the "problem" as psychiatric, with additional implications for discussing the effect on the family and referral to a psychiatrist, but the clinician should not force the patient and family to confront this just yet.

3. If the family accepts this idea, the internist should proceed with treatment of "depression" by drug therapy, especially because "many of the drugs that treat depression also are very good for pain." Venlafaxine and nortriptyline are ideal for

this purpose. This "medicalization" of the "problem of depression" is often easier to tolerate than addressing it as a "psychological problem." If the patient begins to feel better on the pain regimen and antidepressant therapy, and the family is tolerating these interventions, I would advise the internist to suggest a referral to a psychiatrist as an "expert in this area," who can provide help to the internist with "the medication and the problems." If the family has stuck by the internist thus far, it is more likely that they will accept some further interventions and may even be gratified at the prospect of change, although they may not admit it openly. I would assure the family that this referral does *not* mean that the internist is abandoning them; rather, it should be made clear that the work with the psychiatrist is "collaborative," so the patient and family will feel secure that a medical definition of the issue is still at hand and that the internist wants to remain involved.

4. As the family feels their needs (in general) are supported and met, and as the patient's depression begins to lift and the family realizes there is more to life than pain, the equilibrium becomes much easier to shift. An exploration into the reasons that the patient's family has so readily "bought" into this life plan in the first place will be essential as the psychiatrist moves along, however, or the family's unmet, unrecognized needs will certainly sabotage effective treatment (Payne and Norfleet 1986; Sholevar and Perkel 1990).

Further Caveats

At any stage along this path, the family and patient may need to reject the psychiatric solution. In this case, the internist would continue to work with them, gently prodding them to "expect more out of life," and continuing to try to understand the reasons for their difficulty accepting change, as best as possible within the confines of a busy practice. Referral to a pain clinic at any point in this process would be of great assistance to a busy internist with such a complex situation to manage. And, clearly, if the patient continues to have bona fide pain even during and *after* the family equilibrium has been shifted to more healthy behavior, and the depression has lifted, a referral to a pain clinic would be essential. It is important to note, however, that this option should be reserved for late in the intervention; too early a referral would give the family the message that "that is all there is to it," which as we have seen is not the case!

Conclusion

A clinical situation such as this, ostensibly involving "responsible, functional" people, is in fact a great deal more difficult than it might initially appear. But careful management can have a big payoff: the liberation of a family group of four bright, caring, responsible people who could then have more independent, productive lives.

Summary

In this chapter, expert clinicians have provided valuable insights about the management of chronic pain through their detailed review of the assessment and treatment of four patients. In each case, the experts have emphasized different elements of pain management, describing alternative approaches to complex clinical problems. These case discussions offer an opportunity to apply the principles of pain management in classic presentations, emphasizing fundamental principles of quality patient care, especially the complex dynamics of the doctor-patient relationship in the setting of chronic illness and refractory symptoms, and approaches to negotiating comorbid medical and psychiatric illness. Although such patients are uniquely challenging, they provide wonderful opportunities for interdisciplinary collaboration and rewarding work.

Clearly, the patient with chronic pain evokes strong emotional reactions in clinicians. Psychiatrists are uniquely suited to treat such patients and to aid clinicians in other disciplines in their management. Rapid advances in neurobiology, palliative care, and neuropsychiatry offer the promise of better understanding of the complex interplay of biopsychosocial factors in symptom experience and treatment. Psychiatrists have a special role in the ongoing effort to improve the management of pain and psychological distress. These clinical case discussions show the vital role of psychiatry in the provision of comprehensive patient-centered care. Quality management of chronic pain depends on communication and development of a successful therapeutic relationship, and these experts have described the accomplishment of these goals, giving us important principles to guide future care.

References

American Psychiatric Association: Diagnostic and Statistical Manual of Mental Disorders, 4th Edition. Washington, DC, American Psychiatric Association, 1994

Egbunike IG, Chaffee BJ: Antidepressants in the management of chronic pain syndromes. Pharmcotherapy 10:262–270, 1990

Fisch R, Weakland JH, Segal L: The Tactics of Change: Doing Therapy Briefly. San Francisco, CA, Jossey-Bass, 1982

Goldenberg DL, Mayskly M, Mossey C: A randomized, double-blind crossover trial of fluoxetine and amitriptyline in the treatment of fibromyalgia. Arthritis Rheum 39:1852–1859, 1996

Haase EK, Muskin PR: Difficult patients and patients with personality disorders, in Textbook of Primary Care Medicine, 3rd Edition. Edited by Noble J. St. Louis, MO, Mosby, 2000 (in press)

Max MB: Antidepressant drugs as treatments for chronic pain: efficacy and mechanisms, in Pain and the Brain: From Nociception to Cognition, Vol 22. Edited by Bromm B, Desmedt JE. New York, Raven, 1995, pp 501–515

Payne B, Norfleet MA: Chronic pain and the family: a review. Pain 26:1–22, 1986

Rodvold KA, Meyer J: Drug-food interactions with grapefruit juice. Infect Med 13(10):868, 871–873, 912, 1996

Roth RS, Kamholz BA: Major pain syndromes and chronic pain, in Primary Care Psychiatry. Edited by Knesper DJ, Riba MB, Schwenk TL. Philadelphia, PA, WB Saunders, 1997, pp 268–294

Sholevar GP, Perkel R: Family systems intervention and physical illness. Gen Hosp Psychiatry 12:363–372, 1990

Swerdlow M: Anticonvulsant drugs and chronic pain. Clin Neuropharmacol 7:51–82, 1984

Afterword

Mary Jane Massie, M.D.

The contributors to this monograph intended it to meet the needs of an array of diverse clinicians. It may serve as a refreshing update for the psychiatrist skilled in working with individuals who have pain and comorbid psychiatric illness. Alternatively, it may serve as a practical introduction to pain management for the psychiatrist who has shied away from these patients because of the complexity of the patient's presentation, beliefs that "pain patients" are unmotivated and likely untreatable, and concerns (often unwarranted) about drug dependency and addiction. All psychiatrists, whether clinicians, educators, researchers, or administrators, are advocates for psychiatric patients and the profession of psychiatry; consequently, psychiatrists have an important role in the future study and treatment of pain in children and adults, including the elderly. Psychiatrists' basic clinical training contributes much to their nonpsychiatric colleagues' evaluation and treatment of pain.

Mental health researchers have made numerous contributions to the study of pain. Norton et al. (1999) described the significant growth in publications on chronic pain in the psychological database (PsycLIT) accompanied by a decline in publications referenced in the medical database (MEDLINE) over the past decade as evidence that the traditional biomedical orientation to pain has been expanded to include psychosocial parameters: a significant paradigm shift. Although the accomplishments in and contributions to the study of pain by many psychiatrists are substantial, significant research challenges remain. The DSM-IV pain disorder diagnosis still embodies the mind-body dualism that is increasingly viewed as an unhelpful or pejorative distinction in patients with pain (American Psychiatric Association 1994). Surely, this difficult topic will be reconsidered in future nosologies as more evidence is accumulated. Although few studies of the effectiveness of psychotherapeutic interventions for pain have been done

(Norton et al. 1999), an incongruity between what is available technologically and known therapeutically and what is practiced clinically persists (Walco et al. 1994).

The National Institutes of Health (NIH) Technology Assessment Panel on the Integration of Behavioral and Relaxation Approaches Into the Treatment of Chronic Pain and Insomnia (1996), which included psychiatrists as participants of the 12-member nonadvocate multidisciplinary working group, reviewed meta-analyses of the effectiveness of multimodal treatments of pain in clinical settings and described directions for research. The panel found strong evidence for the use of relaxation in the treatment of chronic pain and moderate evidence for the effectiveness of cognitive-behavioral techniques and biofeedback. The panel's following suggestions for research should guide psychiatrists as we move ahead in this new millennium:

- Studies of the mechanism of action and of the efficacy, effectiveness, and cost-effectiveness of behavioral interventions in pain
- Qualitative research to examine the patient's experience of pain
- Research into cross-cultural areas, because values and beliefs about pain are shaped by culture
- Consideration of the effect of race, sex, age, and socioeconomic status on treatment efficacy
- Research on chronic pain treated pharmacologically compared with pain treated behaviorally and on chronic pain treated with combined psychosocial and pharmacological therapy (NIH Technology Assessment Panel 1996)

Finally, the panel addressed the appropriate integration of behavioral and relaxation approaches into health care. Behavioral and psychiatric interventions are costly and time-consuming and are predicated on the willingness and cooperation of the patient. Insurance companies are reluctant to reimburse for psychosocial interventions in general and to reimburse multiple providers for simultaneous treatment (as in a multidisciplinary pain treatment center) of a chronic condition (Gallagher 1999). Results of studies that show which practitioners are the most qualified to provide behavioral interventions in efficacious and cost-effective ways are essential to arm clinicians and administrators with evidence as they negotiate with health insurers and regulatory agencies (NIH Technology Assessment Panel 1996; Stieg et al. 1999). We, as clinicians and members of our professional organization, have clear challenges as we attempt to educate ourselves, our students, our patients, and reimbursement agencies about the effective treatments of pain and to eliminate the barriers to high-quality care for the patient with pain and comorbid psychiatric illness.

References

American Psychiatric Association: Diagnostic and Statistical Manual of Mental Disorders, 4th Edition. Washington, DC, American Psychiatric Association, 1994

Gallagher RM: Primary cancer and pain medicine. Med Clin North Am 83:555–583, 1999

NIH Technology Assessment Panel on Integration of Behavioral and Relaxation Approaches Into the Treatment of Chronic Pain and Insomnia: Integration of behavioral and relaxation approaches into the treatment of chronic pain and insomnia. JAMA 276:313–318, 1996

Norton PJ, Asmundson GJG, Norton GR, et al: Growing pain: 10-year research trends in the study of chronic pain and headache. Pain 79:59–65, 1999

Stieg RL, Lippe P, Shepard TA: Roadblocks to effective pain treatment. Med Clin North Am 83:809–821, 1999

Walco GA, Cassidy RC, Schechter NL: Pain, hurt, and harm: the ethics of pain control in infants and children. N Engl J Med 331:541–544, 1994

Index

*Page numbers printed in **boldface** type refer to tables or figures.*

Bone pain arising from osseous metastases, 15
Brachial plexus, injury to, 13
Brain stem tractotomies, **65**
Brain stimulation, 67
Breast cancer treatment, nerve injury following, amitriptyline and, 30
Buprenorphine, 58
Burns, 5
Bursitis, 5

Caffeine, 45
Calcitonin, 44
Cancer pain, 1, 5–6
  opioids in management of, 53–57
  undertreatment, 53
Capsaicin, 43
Carbamazepine, **37,** 140
Carisoprodol, 42
Carpal tunnel syndrome, 16
Catastrophizing, reducing, 162
Causalgia, 16
Celecoxib, **25**
Central nervous system
  lesions of, 13
  prostaglandin inhibition in, 24
Central pain syndromes, 6, 110
Cervical strain, 5
Chemical neurolysis, 62–63
Chemical rhizotomy, 62
Chemical stimuli, 2
Chemotherapy-induced stomatitis, 6
Childhood sexual abuse, chronic pelvic pain, 104–105
Chlorphenesin carbamate, 42
Chlorzoxazone, 42
Choline magnesium trisalicylate, **25**

Chronic pain. *See also* specific types of pain
  associated with nonprogressive organic lesion, **9,** 6–7
  biopsychosocial model, schematic, **4**
  definition of, 2–3
  low back pain, 98–99
  models of, 3–4, **4**
  nonmalignant pain syndrome, usage of term, 17
  pelvic, 110
  of unknown etiology, 7, 17
  tension headache, 7, 17
Cingulotomy, **65**
Cirrhosis, contraindication in analgesic therapy, 26
Clomipramine, 31, 32
Clonazepam, 38, 45
Clonidine, 33
Codeine, 55
Cognitive-behavioral strategies, 162
Cognitive-evaluative dimension of pain, 3
Communication, with patient, importance of, 141
Compensation, pain-related, patients receiving, 113
Constipation, from opioids, management of, 49, **51**
Contingency management, 112
Control, perceived, enhancing, 162
Conversion pain disorder, 90, 102
Cordotomy
  open, **65**
  percutaneous, **65**
Cortical changes, phantom limb pain from, 95

Pain modulation, mounted by neural activity, 95–97

Pancreas, injury to, 15

Parental neglect, 145–146, 148

Paroxetine, 31, 140, 156, 157

Pathophysiology, inferred, 15–17

Patients with pain, categories of, 4–7

Pelvic pain, 104–105, 110
  sexual abuse, 104–105
  of unknown etiology, 7, 17

Perceived control, enhancing, 162

Perforation of GI tract, NSAID-related, 27

Peripheral afferents, sensitization of, 95

Personality disorder, severe, 18

Pes anserine bursitis, 5

Phantom limb pain
  calcitonin for, 44
  from cortical changes, 95

Phenoxybenzamine, 44

Phenytoin, **37**

Physical dependence on opioids, 52

Pimozide, 45

Piroxicam, **25,** 27

Polyneuropathy, 13
  painful, 6

Postcordotomy dysesthesia, central pain syndrome, 66

Postherpetic neuralgia, 6, 33, 110
  amitriptyline for, 30
  desipramine for, 31

Postoperative pain, 33

Potassium ions, 2

Prazosin, 44

Prescription drugs, history of use, 19

Progressive medical diseases, chronic pain due to, 6

Propionic acids, **25**

Propoxyphene, 55

Propranolol, 44

Prostaglandin, 2
  inhibition in central nervous system, 24

Psychoanalytic theory of psychogenic pain, 102

Psychodynamic model, 102–106

Psychogenic headache, doxepin for, 31

Psychogenic pain, 16, 90
  diagnosis of, 90–92
  physiological sources of, 94–101
  psychoanalytic theory, 102
  psychological causation, 92–94
  usage of term, 91

Psychological approaches to pain, 67–68
  behavior therapy, 68
  biofeedback, 68
  distraction techniques, 68
  exercise program, 68
  hypnosis, 68
  relaxation training, 68

Psychological causation, psychogenic pain disorder, 92–94

Psychological disturbance, pain associated with, 7

Psychological models, 102–111

Psychosocial functioning, assessment of, 18

Radiographic procedures, 14

Rapport with patient, establishment of, 161–162

Recurrent acute pain, 5

Weakness, 18
WHO (World Health
    Organization), analgesic
    ladder approach, **54, 57,**
    53–56
Withdrawal, from opioids, 52

World Health Organization
    (WHO), analgesic ladder
    approach, **54, 57,** 53–56
Writhing, acute pain with, 9

Zimelidine, 31